UNDERSTANDING CHILDHOOD EPILEPSY & SEIZURES:
A Guide for Parents.

By
Cynthia E. Cortez.

TABLE OF CONTENTS

CHAPTER 1

<u>Seizing Moments: Understanding Childhood Epilepsy & Seizures</u>

The history of epilepsy and seizures in children extends back to ancient times, with numerous cultural beliefs and medical developments affecting our knowledge of this neurological illness. Epilepsy is characterized by repeated seizures, which are aberrant electrical discharges in the brain that result in momentary interruptions in normal brain function. Seizures in children may be a tough condition, impacting their development, schooling, and general quality of life.

In ancient cultures, epilepsy was typically perceived through a supernatural perspective. People thought that seizures were caused by malevolent spirits, curses, or divine retribution. Treatments varied from exorcisms and religious ceremonies to charms and amulets. These ancient cultures had inadequate medical knowledge and lacked the instruments to appreciate the complicated nature of epilepsy.

The ancient Greeks, however, made substantial advances in understanding epilepsy. The Greek physician Hippocrates, long regarded as the founder of modern medicine, rejected the concept of epilepsy as a supernatural phenomena.

He understood that seizures originated in the brain and suggested a more reasonable explanation. Hippocrates regarded epilepsy as a "sacred disease" and distanced it from religious ideas. This change in thinking created the framework for a scientific approach to epilepsy.

Despite these early breakthroughs, beliefs regarding epilepsy lingered through the Middle Ages and the Renaissance. Epileptic persons were typically ostracized and marginalized, with many being deemed possessed or mentally sick. The lack of knowledge led to prejudice and maltreatment.

In the 19th century, tremendous progress was achieved in the area of epilepsy. The French physician Jean-Martin Charcot conducted comprehensive clinical observations and categorised numerous forms of seizures.

He also identified the relationship between epilepsy and other neurological illnesses. Charcot's findings established the framework for subsequent scientific investigation and helped separate epilepsy from other illnesses with similar symptoms.

In the early 20th century, developments in electroencephalography (EEG) changed the diagnosis and understanding of epilepsy. The EEG permitted the recording and study of brain waves, offering vital insights into the electrical activity of the brain during seizures. This finding led to the creation of antiepileptic medicines (AEDs) in the 1930s. Phenobarbital was the first successful AED, followed by additional drugs like phenytoin and carbamazepine.

Over time, the medical profession came to acknowledge the special issues of epilepsy in children. Pediatric epileptologists concentrate on studying the unique forms of seizures and syndromes that afflict children, as well as their influence on development and cognition. They also devised particular therapeutic techniques and treatments to target the unique requirements of pediatric patients.

In recent decades, developments in imaging technology, like magnetic resonance imaging (MRI), have offered more insights into the structural and functional problems associated with epilepsy. This has enabled for more exact diagnosis and better treatment regimens, including surgical possibilities for drug-resistant instances.

Today, the care of epilepsy and seizures in children entails a multidisciplinary approach. Pediatric neurologists, epileptologists, neuropsychologists, and other healthcare specialists cooperate to offer comprehensive treatment. Treatment options include medication, nutritional therapy (e.g., ketogenic diet), neurostimulation methods (e.g., vagus nerve stimulation), and, in certain instances, epilepsy surgery.

Despite great improvement, epilepsy in children remains a complicated disorder with continuing issues. Research continues to find the underlying processes, hereditary variables, and possibly novel therapy routes. Efforts to promote awareness, decrease stigma, and give support to afflicted children and their families are crucial to enhancing their quality of life.

In conclusion, the history of epilepsy and seizures in children has progressed from ancient beliefs to present scientific knowledge. From the early ideas of demonic possession to the awareness of the brain's involvement in seizure activity, breakthroughs in medical knowledge, diagnosis, and therapy have offered hope to many youngsters living with epilepsy. Ongoing research and compassionate treatment will significantly advance our knowledge and management of this illness, increasing outcomes and quality of life for children with epilepsy.

WHAT ARE CHILDHOOD EPILEPSY & SEIZURES

Childhood epilepsy is a neurological condition that affects children and is characterized by recurring seizures. Seizures occur when there is a rapid and abnormal burst of electrical activity in the brain. These episodes may induce a range of symptoms, depending on the part of the brain affected and the intensity of the seizure.

Seizures may be categorized into two primary categories: focal seizures and generalized seizures. Focal seizures, also known as partial seizures, occur when the aberrant electrical activity is localized to a single portion of the brain.

This may induce a number of symptoms, such as muscular twitching, alterations in sensation, or altered awareness. On the other hand, generalized seizures include aberrant electrical activity over the whole brain and may induce loss of consciousness, convulsions, and stiffness or shaking of the body.

Childhood epilepsy may have numerous causes. Sometimes, it might be connected to hereditary issues, meaning that it runs in families. Other times, it might be caused by brain abnormalities, such as malformations or lesions. In certain situations, epilepsy may be a consequence of brain damage caused by infections, head traumas, or other medical disorders.

If your kid has been diagnosed with epilepsy, it's crucial to recognize that they are not alone. Epilepsy is one of the most prevalent neurological illnesses in children, and it may afflict children of various ages and backgrounds. It's also crucial to realize that having epilepsy does not define your kid or restrict their potential. With the correct care and support, most children with epilepsy may live full and active lives.

Managing pediatric epilepsy entails working closely with healthcare specialists, including neurologists and epileptologists. They will assist select the proper treatment strategy for your kid. Treatment options may include antiepileptic drugs, lifestyle adjustments, and in certain situations, surgical treatments. The objective of therapy is to manage seizures while reducing negative effects and increasing the child's quality of life.

As a parent, it may be tough to observe your kid suffering seizures. During a seizure, it's vital to be cool and guarantee the child's safety. You may gently move them away from possible risks, such as sharp items or harsh surfaces. It's normally advisable to time the seizure length and notice any special aspects that might aid healthcare experts in their examination.

In addition to medical care, there are actions you may do at home to assist your child's well-being. Encouraging a healthy lifestyle, such as establishing regular sleep patterns, having a balanced diet, and participating in physical exercise, may help minimize the frequency and severity of seizures. It's also crucial to establish a safe environment by eliminating possible risks and teaching family members, teachers, and other caregivers about epilepsy and how to react during a seizure.

While childhood epilepsy may be tough for both children and their families, it's crucial to stay cheerful and hopeful. With the correct therapy and care, many children with epilepsy see a considerable decrease in seizures over time, and some may even outgrow the disease.
Remember to seek out support groups, organizations, and other families who have experience with epilepsy. Connecting with individuals who understand your position may give essential emotional support and practical help.

In conclusion, infantile epilepsy is a neurological condition marked by recurring seizures. It may have many reasons and affects children of all ages. With adequate medical care, lifestyle adaptations, and support, most children with epilepsy may enjoy meaningful lives. It's crucial to work closely with healthcare providers, establish a secure atmosphere, and seek support from those who have experience with epilepsy. Remember that you are not alone on this path, and there is aid available to handle the obstacles of childhood epilepsy.

WHY DO SEIZURES AND EPILEPSY OCCUR IN CHILDREN?

In the domain of pediatric neurology, few illnesses inspire as much fascination and anxiety as seizures and epilepsy. These mysterious illnesses, defined by aberrant electrical activity in the brain, may substantially impair the lives of children and their families.

Seizures, frequently the defining manifestation of epilepsy, may appear as an unanticipated variety of physical and behavioral symptoms, leading to a cascade of inquiries and worries. Delving into the delicate workings of the young brain, this essay tries to shed light on the reasons and processes of seizures and epilepsy in children, allowing us to better understand and assist these little fighters.

I. The Brain's Electrical Symphony:
To appreciate the development of seizures and epilepsy, it is necessary to fathom the incredible intricacy of the brain's electrical circuitry. Our brains are a symphony of communication between billions of neurons, which depend on perfectly timed electrical impulses to transfer information. These impulses form a choreographed dance of coordinated activity, needed for appropriate brain function.

II. Unraveling the Mystery of Seizures:
Seizures are the outcome of an electrical storm, shattering the brain's fragile homeostasis. When neurons fire in an aberrant, excessive, or disordered fashion, they create a burst of electrical activity that appears as seizures. While seizures may be an indication of several underlying

disorders, epilepsy is diagnosed when a kid suffers recurring, unprovoked seizures.

III. The Multifaceted Causes of Seizures and Epilepsy in Children:
Understanding the causes of seizures and epilepsy in children entails navigating a diverse terrain. While many instances remain idiopathic, some events have been identified as probable triggers:

a) Genetic Factors: In certain situations, a child's genetic composition might play a vital role in the development of seizures and epilepsy. Various gene alterations have been implicated, impacting ion channels, neurotransmitters, and cellular signaling pathways involved in neural transmission.

b) Structural Abnormalities: Congenital deformities of the brain, such as cortical dysplasia, neuronal migration problems, or tumors, may alter normal brain circuitry and trigger seizures

c) Perinatal Factors: Complications during pregnancy and delivery, such as maternal infections, prenatal medication exposure, or oxygen deprivation, may lead to an increased risk of seizures and epilepsy in children.

d) illnesses: Certain illnesses, such as meningitis, encephalitis, or even high fevers, may provoke seizures, especially in young children with underdeveloped immune systcms.

e) Metabolic abnormalities: In rare situations, inborn errors of metabolism, such as mitochondrial abnormalities or problems affecting amino acid metabolism, may lead to seizures and epilepsy.

f) Traumatic Brain Injury: Head trauma, either due to accidents or non-accidental traumas, may cause structural damage to the brain, resulting in seizures.

IV. Understanding the Epileptic Network:
The brain's complicated network of linked neurons may create an "epileptic network" in certain youngsters. This network comprises faulty connections and heightened excitability in particular brain areas, predisposing patients to repeated seizures. These regions may vary from restricted locations, known as focal seizures, to encompass both hemispheres of the brain, called generalized seizures.

V. Diagnosis and Treatment:
Accurate diagnosis is critical for efficient therapy of seizures and epilepsy in children. Detailed medical history, physical examination, and diagnostic procedures such as electroencephalogram (EEG), magnetic resonance imaging (MRI), and genetic testing are performed to discover the underlying cause and select the most effective treatment plan. Treatment options may include antiepileptic drugs, dietary therapy (such as the ketogenic diet),

neurostimulation devices, or, in some situations, epilepsy surgery.

Conclusion:
Seizures and epilepsy in children are complicated neurological diseases with diverse underlying causes. Understanding the elements that lead to their growth enables for improved diagnosis, treatment, and management measures. By extending our understanding and fostering research in this sector, we get closer to improving the lives of children afflicted by seizures and epilepsy, giving them the care, support, and opportunities they need.

WHAT TRIGGERS A SEIZURE IN CHILDREN?

Seizures may be an unpleasant experience for both children and their parents. Understanding the triggers and causes of seizures is vital for parents to appropriately manage their child's condition. In this thorough guide, we will discuss the numerous causes that might induce seizures in children, along with measures to decrease their recurrence and protect the well-being of your kid.

Common Triggers for Seizures in Children:
1. Sleep Deprivation:
Lack of proper sleep or irregular sleep patterns might provoke seizures in youngsters. Ensuring your kid maintains a normal sleep regimen, gets adequate restorative sleep, and avoids sleep deficit is vital.

2. Stress and Emotional Factors:
Emotional stress, worry, or great enthusiasm might function as triggers for seizures. Helping your kid handle stress via relaxation methods, therapy, and fostering a supportive atmosphere might be useful.

3. Fever:
Febrile seizures are quite frequent in young children and are commonly induced by high

temperatures. It is vital to treat your child's fever quickly by delivering appropriate fever-reducing drugs and employing cooling measures, such as lukewarm baths or sponging.

4. Sensory Overload:
Bright, flashing lights, loud sounds, and excessive sensory stimulation may provoke seizures in certain youngsters. Minimizing exposure to these triggers and providing a quiet, calming atmosphere may lower the likelihood of seizures.

5. Missed Medications:
If your kid has been taking antiepileptic drugs, skipping doses or unusual medication regimens might increase the probability of seizures. Adhering to the specified drug schedule is vital to maintain seizure control.

6. Illness and Infections:
Certain conditions, such as respiratory infections or gastrointestinal problems,

might reduce the seizure threshold in vulnerable children. Maintaining appropriate hygiene standards, adopting a healthy lifestyle, and swiftly addressing any underlying conditions will help lessen the risk.

7. Fluctuations in Blood Sugar Levels:
Significant variations in blood sugar levels, such as hypoglycemia (low blood sugar) or hyperglycemia (high blood sugar), may provoke seizures. Ensuring your kid follows a well-balanced diet, eats meals at regular intervals, and checks blood sugar levels (if required) might be useful.

8. Hormonal Changes:
Hormonal changes during puberty or the menstrual cycle might increase the frequency of seizures in certain youngsters. Keeping note of any trends connected to hormonal swings and working closely with your child's healthcare professional may help manage these seizures successfully.

Management and Support:
To treat seizures properly, it is vital to engage closely with your child's healthcare team. Some techniques that may benefit seizure control include:

1. Creating a Seizure Action Plan:
Developing a detailed seizure action plan with your child's healthcare practitioner will give information on seizure treatment throughout different scenarios. This plan should contain emergency contacts, prescription instructions, and recommended procedures to follow during a seizure.

2. Medication Adherence:
Administering antiepileptic drugs as recommended by the healthcare professional is vital. Regularly check and renew medications to avoid any changes in pharmaceutical treatment.

3. Lifestyle Modifications:

Encourage your kid to develop a healthy lifestyle by fostering frequent exercise, a balanced diet, and stress-reducing hobbies. Avoiding excessive coffee and keeping hydrated are also suggested.

4. Recognizing and Avoiding Triggers:
Identify particular factors that may contribute to seizures in your kid and take necessary precautions to reduce their exposure. For example, if flashing lights induce seizures, avoid places with strobe lights or quick visual stimulation.

5. Educating Others:
Ensure that family members, caretakers, teachers, and other others engaged in your child's life are taught about epilepsy, seizures, and the proper reaction during an episode. This insight may help establish a supportive and safe environment for your kid.

Conclusion:

Understanding the triggers and causes of seizures in children is vital for parents to appropriately manage their child's condition. By applying proper techniques, such as supporting healthy lifestyles, controlling stress, and avoiding recognized triggers, parents may greatly minimize the incidence and effect of seizures. Working closely with healthcare providers and having open communication will guarantee thorough support for your child's well-being. Remember, every kid is unique, and tailored care and attention are crucial to effectively controlling seizures.

DIAGNOSIS & TREATMENT OF CHILDHOOD EPILEPSY AND SEIZURE

Epilepsy and seizures may be tough for both children and their parents to live with. Understanding the diagnosis and treatment choices is vital for managing the disease properly. In this part, we will discuss the process of diagnosing epilepsy and seizures in children, as well as several treatment techniques available to give the best care and support for your kid.

DIAGNOSIS:
Diagnosing epilepsy and seizures in children necessitates a full assessment by a healthcare specialist, generally a pediatric neurologist or epileptologist. The diagnostic method generally involves the following steps:

1. Medical History: The doctor will evaluate your child's medical history, including any documented seizure events, their frequency, length, and related symptoms. They will also enquire about any family history of epilepsy or other neurological problems.

2. Physical Examination: A comprehensive physical examination will be undertaken to check your child's general health, and neurological development, and search for

any physical indications or anomalies that may aid with the diagnosis.

3. Electroencephalogram (EEG): An EEG is a non-invasive test that monitors the electrical activity of the brain. Your kid will have electrodes implanted on their head, and their brain waves will be recorded. This test may assist uncover aberrant brain activity that may be symptomatic of epilepsy.

4. Imaging Tests: Imaging tests, such as magnetic resonance imaging (MRI) or computed tomography (CT), may be conducted to discover any structural abnormalities or brain lesions that might be causing the seizures.

5. Blood Tests: Blood tests may be undertaken to look for any underlying metabolic or genetic problems that might be connected with seizures.

6. Video EEG Monitoring: In certain circumstances, a prolonged video EEG monitoring may be essential. This includes monitoring brain activity for a lengthy time, generally 24-48 hours, to catch any aberrant electrical patterns linked with seizures.

TREATMENT:

Once the diagnosis of epilepsy or seizures is established, the following step is to select an effective treatment strategy. The choice of therapy will depend on various aspects, including the kind of seizures, their frequency and intensity, the child's age, general health, and any underlying problems. The following are frequent therapeutic techniques for children with epilepsy:

1. Medicines: Anti-seizure medicines, often known as antiepileptic drugs (AEDs), are the most prevalent therapeutic choice. These drugs assist control or minimize the frequency and severity of seizures. The

doctor will prescribe the most suited medicine based on your child's individual requirements and frequent monitoring will be necessary to modify the dose and manage any possible adverse effects.

2. Ketogenic Diet: In certain situations, a ketogenic diet may be advised for children with epilepsy, particularly if seizures are not well-controlled with medication alone. This high-fat, low-carbohydrate diet may help decrease seizure activity in certain children, however, it needs rigorous adherence and frequent supervision by a healthcare practitioner.

3. Vagus Nerve Stimulation (VNS): VNS is a surgical therapeutic option for children with epilepsy who do not react well to medicines. A tiny device is implanted beneath the skin, generally in the chest region, which provides electrical impulses to the brain via the vagus nerve, helping to minimize seizure activity.

4. Responsive Neurostimulation (RNS): RNS is another surgical therapy option that includes implanting a device in the brain to detect aberrant electrical activity and give tailored electrical stimulation to avoid seizures.

5. Epilepsy Surgery: In some circumstances, where seizures originate from a particular region of the brain that may be safely removed without causing major harm, epilepsy surgery may be explored. This approach is generally reserved for children with seizures that are not well-controlled with drugs and who have a distinct seizure focal.

Diagnosing and treating epilepsy and seizures in children involves a comprehensive approach encompassing medical history, physical exams, diagnostic testing, and tailored treatment strategies. By working together with healthcare specialists, parents may play a significant part in controlling their child's illness and providing them with essential support and care. It is essential to remember that every child's path with epilepsy is unique, and with the correct treatment and continued care, many children may have satisfying lives.

EXPLAINING TO YOUR CHILD HOW THE BRAIN WORKS AND WHY SEIZURES HAPPEN

As parents, it is normal to be anxious when our children encounter seizures. Explaining the workings of the brain and why seizures occur may help reduce anxieties and establish a basis for improved knowledge. In this part, we will investigate the complexity of the brain, its numerous activities, and how seizures might appear. By breaking down difficult issues into simple words, we can empower both parents and children to confront seizures with understanding and empathy.

1. The Marvels of the Brain:
The brain is an extraordinary organ that regulates everything we do, think, and feel. It is like a supercomputer that organizes our body's operations, enabling us to move, communicate, and see the world around us. The brain is made up of billions of nerve cells called neurons, which are responsible for delivering and receiving information throughout the body.

2. The Parts of the Brain:
To comprehend seizures, it's vital to have a fundamental grasp of the brain's primary parts:

a) Cerebrum: This is the biggest region of the brain and is responsible for thinking, learning, and regulating voluntary motions. It is split into two hemispheres, the left and right, each governing the opposing side of the body.

b) Cerebellum: Located near the rear of the brain, the cerebellum aids with coordination, balance, and muscular control.

c) Brainstem: Connecting the brain to the spinal cord, the brainstem governs critical activities including breathing, heartbeat, and sleep.

3. Neurons and Electrical Signals:
Neurons connect with each other via electrical impulses, which enable information to pass throughout the brain and body. These impulses are like small sparks that speed across the neurons, transporting information from one section of the brain to another.

4. What Happens During a Seizure:
Sometimes, the brain's electrical impulses get interrupted, leading to a seizure. Imagine the brain's electrical activity as a symphony where each instrument performs

in harmony. During a seizure, there is an abrupt spike of electrical activity that breaks this equilibrium, leading the brain's signals to become jumbled.

5. Different Types of Seizures:
Seizures may show in numerous ways, depending on the area of the brain afflicted. Some typical forms of seizures include:

a) Generalized Seizures: These affect both sides of the brain simultaneously, resulting in loss of consciousness, muscular stiffness, convulsions, or jerking motions.

b) Focal Seizures: These occur in a particular region of the brain and may induce strange feelings, emotions, or repeated movements in a single section of the body.

6. Triggers and Seizure Control:
Seizures may be provoked by different reasons, such as sleep deprivation, stress,

particular meals, or flashing lights. It is crucial for both children and parents to be aware of possible triggers and take necessary actions to limit the risk of seizures.

7. How Seizures are Treated:
If a kid is diagnosed with epilepsy, a disorder marked by repeated seizures, there are numerous therapeutic options available. Medications may be provided to control or lessen the frequency of seizures. In rare circumstances, physicians may offer various therapy, such as dietary modifications or surgery, to control seizures efficiently.

Conclusion:
Understanding how the brain works and explaining seizures to your kid may build a feeling of empowerment and minimize worry. By breaking down complicated subjects into smaller words, you may offer your kid with the information and assistance they need. Remember, open

communication, patience, and empathy are vital when addressing seizures with your kid. Encourage them to ask questions, and seek expert help from physicians or support groups to ensure you have the resources you need on this journey together.

GUIDANCE FOR PARENTS FOLLOWING THEIR CHILD'S SINGLE SEIZURE

As a parent, knowing that your kid has undergone a seizure may be a frightening and bewildering experience. It is vital to be calm and helpful throughout this period.

Understanding The Seizure:
1. Reassurance: It is crucial to reassure your kid that they are secure and that you are there to help them. Emphasize that suffering a seizure does not define them as a person and that it does not necessarily imply they have epilepsy.

2. Medical Evaluation: Contact a healthcare professional promptly after the seizure. Describe the seizure in full, including the length, appearance, and any other noteworthy observations. Your kid may be sent to a neurologist or an epilepsy specialist for further examination.

3. Document the Event: Keep a record of the seizure, including the date, time, and length. Document any odd behavior, movements, or symptoms witnessed before, during, or after the seizure. This information will be essential during medical consultations.

4. Seizure Triggers: Discuss with your kid whether they recall anything unexpected or out of the norm before the seizure. Identifying probable causes, such as lack of sleep, stress, or specific meals, might aid in controlling future episodes.

5. Safety Precautions: Ensure your child's safety during and after a seizure. Clear the

immediate surroundings of any things that may provide a danger of harm. Avoid limiting your child's movements, and instead, gently lead them away from harmful situations. Placing something soft beneath their head might give extra padding.

Medical Consultation:
1. Medical History: Prepare a full medical history for your kid, including past illnesses, injuries, medicines, and family history of seizures or epilepsy. This information will aid the healthcare expert in assessing the reason and proper treatment approach.

2. Diagnostic testing: The healthcare expert may offer diagnostic testing to better understand the underlying cause of the seizure. These tests may include blood testing, an electroencephalogram (EEG), brain imaging (MRI or CT scan), or other specialist examinations.

3. Seek Clarification: Do not hesitate to raise questions during medical visits. Seek clarification on any medical jargon, test procedures, or treatment alternatives that you may not completely understand. It is crucial to have a comprehensive grasp of your child's condition and the suggested course of treatment.

4. Medication and Treatment Options: Depending on the result of the diagnostic tests and medical examination, your child's healthcare expert may prescribe drugs to prevent future seizures. Understand the advantages, possible adverse effects, and correct administration of the prescription drug. Discuss other therapy choices, if available, and any lifestyle alterations that may be useful.

Supporting Your Child:
1. Emotional Support: Remain open, sensitive, and understanding towards your child's emotional needs. Encourage open

communication and enable them to share their thoughts, anxieties, and concerns. Reassure them that you are there to help them during the trip.

2. Educate and Normalize: Equip yourself with information about seizures, epilepsy, and related issues. Share age-appropriate information with your kid, their siblings, and other family members to help them understand and support their sibling or friend.

3. School and Social Support: Notify your child's school about the seizure incident and train teachers and staff members on how to react in case of a seizure. Foster a supportive and inclusive atmosphere for your kid at school and in social situations.

4. Lifestyle Factors: Encourage your kid to keep a healthy lifestyle by ensuring regular sleep patterns, stress management, and a balanced food. Adequate relaxation, stress

reduction measures, and a good diet may help lessen the frequency and severity of seizures in certain circumstances.

Conclusion:

Experiencing a seizure may be stressful for both you and your kid. However, by getting proper medical treatment, knowing the nature of the seizure, and offering emotional support, you can successfully assist your kid through this experience. Remember, each kid's condition is unique, and regular contact with healthcare specialists will be crucial in delivering the best possible treatment for your child.

EXPLORING THE DIFFERENT TYPES OF SEIZURES AND THEIR RESPECTIVE TREATMENTS

Seizures are a frequent neurological condition affecting individuals of all ages, including children. Understanding the various forms of seizures and their therapies is vital for parents to help their children properly. In recent years, there has been a movement from the previous method of seizure categorization to a new approach, which gives a more thorough knowledge of seizures. Let's look into the old and modern categorization systems, along with their corresponding treatments.

Old Classification System:
In the past, seizures were largely categorized into two primary categories: generalized seizures and partial seizures.

Generalized Seizures:
Generalized seizures include aberrant electrical activity on both sides of the brain. They may be further classified into subtypes:

a) Absence Seizures: Absence seizures, also known as petit mal seizures, are prevalent in youngsters. They commonly present as short spells of staring, transient loss of consciousness, and unresponsiveness. These convulsions normally persist for a few seconds and may go undetected. Treatment generally requires drugs like ethosuximide or valproic acid.

b) Tonic-Clonic Seizures: Tonic-clonic seizures, previously termed grand mal seizures, are characterized by abrupt loss of consciousness, and bodily rigidity (tonic phase), followed by jerking movements (clonic phase). After the seizure, the individual may suffer bewilderment and weariness. Medications like valproic acid, lamotrigine, or carbamazepine are routinely administered.

c) Myoclonic Seizures: Myoclonic seizures feature quick, short, and fast muscular jerks. These jerks might affect individual muscle groups or the whole body. Medications such as valproic acid, levetiracetam, or clonazepam are commonly used for therapy.

d) Atonic Seizures: Atonic seizures, often termed drop attacks, involve abrupt loss of muscular tone, resulting in falls or drop episodes. Treatment may require drugs like lamotrigine, valproic acid, or levetiracetam.

Partial Seizures:
Partial seizures, also known as focal seizures, originate in a localized region of the brain and may or may not include loss of consciousness. They may be further classified as follows:

a) Simple Partial Seizures: Simple partial seizures do not induce loss of consciousness. They may result in odd feelings, jerking movements, or tingling in certain body areas. Antiepileptic medicines (AEDs) such as carbamazepine, oxcarbazepine, or phenytoin are commonly recommended.

b) Complex Partial Seizures: Complex partial seizures generally entail abnormalities in consciousness or awareness. The individual may display repeated actions, bewilderment, or unresponsiveness during the seizure. Medications like carbamazepine, lamotrigine, or levetiracetam are routinely utilized.

New Classification System:
To give a more complete knowledge of seizures, the International League Against Epilepsy (ILAE) created a new categorization system in 2017. This method classifies seizures depending on their onset and the brain areas involved. It comprises of three primary categories:

Focal Onset Seizures:
Formerly known as partial seizures, focal onset seizures develop in a particular region of the brain. They may be further differentiated depending on whether the individual retains consciousness (aware focal onset seizures) or has altered awareness (impaired awareness focal onset

seizures). Treatment methods vary on the exact kind of seizure and may entail drugs, lifestyle adjustments, and even surgical intervention.

Generalized Onset Seizures:
Generalized onset seizures include both sides of the brain from the outset. They may be further split into six categories, including absence, tonic, clonic, myoclonic, atonic, and tonic-clonic seizures. Treatment options include antiepileptic drugs customized to the individual seizure type, lifestyle adjustments, and possibly surgical treatments for select instances.

Unknown Onset Seizures:
This category is utilized when the actual commencement of a seizure is uncertain or when there is inadequate evidence to define it effectively. Further diagnostic tests and assessments may be required to establish the optimal therapy strategy.

Treatment Options:
The treatment of seizures seeks to lessen the frequency and severity of seizures while reducing negative effects. The choice of therapy relies on the seizure type, individual variables, and the underlying cause of the seizures. Common treatment options include:

Antiepileptic Medications: These medications are often the first line of therapy for most seizure types. They function by stabilizing aberrant electrical activity in the brain. Examples of regularly administered antiepileptic drugs include carbamazepine, valproic acid, lamotrigine, and levetiracetam.

Ketogenic Diet: In certain situations, a ketogenic diet, which is rich in fat and low in carbs, may be advised, especially for children with drug-resistant seizures. This diet replicates the metabolic state of fasting and has demonstrated favorable results in lowering seizure frequency.

Vagus Nerve Stimulation (VNS): VNS includes the implantation of a device that stimulates the vagus nerve in the neck. This therapy may help decrease seizure frequency and intensity, especially in those who do not react well to medicines.

Surgery: In some circumstances, surgery may be considered to remove the brain tissue responsible for initiating seizures. This technique is often investigated when seizures are resistant to medicine and originate from a particular location of the brain.

It's crucial for parents to contact healthcare specialists knowledgeable in managing seizures to find the most suitable treatment strategy for their kid. Regular monitoring, compliance with medicines, and a supportive environment are vital in controlling seizures efficiently and boosting the overall well-being of the kid.

EPISODES THAT ARE USUALLY MISTAKEN FOR SEIZURES IN KIDS

As parents, it's crucial to be aware of numerous health risks that might impact our children. Sometimes, certain incidents or actions in children might be misinterpreted for seizures, creating fear and uncertainty. However, it's crucial to remember that not all occurrences mimic seizures, and recognizing the distinctions may help soothe parental anxiety. In this post, we will cover frequent episodes that are commonly mistaken for seizures in children, clarifying their features and giving recommendations on whether to seek medical assistance.

Breath-Holding Spells:
Breath-holding spells are instances when a youngster holds their breath involuntarily, generally in reaction to anger, irritation, or

pain. These episodes are more prevalent in toddlers and are not seizures. During a breath-holding period, the youngster may grow pale or blue, lose consciousness, and momentarily cease breathing. This might be scary for parents, but it is vital to stay cool.

Differentiating Features:
- Breath-holding episodes often last less than one minute, but seizures frequently last longer.
- Children having breath-holding episodes recover consciousness spontaneously, while seizures are typically followed by a period of disorientation or lethargy.
- Breath-holding episodes are often caused by particular emotions or discomfort, but seizures may occur without any apparent reason.

Febrile Seizures:
Febrile seizures are convulsions that may occur with a fever, generally in children

between the ages of 6 months and 5 years. Although they might be alarming, febrile seizures are typically harmless and do not produce long-term repercussions.

Differentiating Features:
- Febrile seizures occur with a sudden increase in body temperature, often exceeding 100.4°F (38°C).
- They generally last less than five minutes and feature jerking or twitching motions of the arms, legs, and face.
- Febrile seizures are not caused by epilepsy and do not suggest a greater chance of having epilepsy later in life.

Night Terrors:
Night terrors, also known as sleep terrors, are bouts of great dread or terror that occur during sleep. These episodes are more prevalent in children aged 3 to 8 years and may be readily misinterpreted for seizures owing to their dramatic character.

Differentiating Features:
- Night terrors often occur throughout the first few hours of sleep during non-REM (rapid eye movement) sleep, but seizures may occur at any moment.
- Children having night terrors may sit up suddenly, scream, and seem to be inconsolable or bewildered, yet they are not receptive to consoling or reassuring remarks.
- Unlike seizures, night terrors do not include aberrant movements or loss of consciousness and are typically not recalled in the morning.

Syncope:
Syncope, commonly referred to as fainting, is a temporary loss of consciousness caused by a temporary decrease in blood flow to the brain. Although it might be scary, syncope is often benign and not related with seizures.

Differentiating Features:

- Syncope is generally preceded by lightheadedness, dizziness, or feeling faint, but seizures often strike quickly without warning.
- During a syncope episode, children normally fall and rapidly recover consciousness, but seizures may be followed by a postictal phase of bewilderment or lethargy.
- Syncope is usually precipitated by conditions such as dehydration, extended standing, or mental stress, but seizures may occur without any known reason.

When to Seek Medical Attention:
While most occurrences mistaken for seizures are typically innocuous, it is vital to see a healthcare expert if:

- The episode lasts more than five minutes.

- The youngster has trouble breathing or goes blue.
- The infant does not recover consciousness soon following the occurrence.
- The youngster endures recurring episodes or seizures run in the family.
- The event is accompanied by additional worrying symptoms including severe headache, vomiting, or strange behavior.

Conclusion:

Recognizing the distinctions between episodes that mimic seizures and genuine seizures is critical for parents. By recognizing the features of breath-holding episodes, febrile seizures, night terrors, and syncope, parents may minimize undue worry and seek proper medical treatment when required. Always see a healthcare expert for a complete examination and diagnosis to guarantee your child's well-being

DO'S & DON'TS WHEN YOUR CHILD IS HAVING A SEIZURE

Seizures may be a terrifying event for both children and parents. As a parent, it is crucial to know how to react and offer the required care when your kid is experiencing a seizure or living with epilepsy. Understanding the do's and don'ts in these scenarios will assist protect the safety and well-being of your kid. Here are some recommendations to follow:

DO'S:

Stay Calm: It's vital to stay calm during a seizure. While watching your kid experiencing a seizure may be frightening, being cool can enable you to give appropriate aid and support.

Ensure Safety: Focus on establishing a safe atmosphere for your youngster. Clear the area of any sharp objects, furniture, or possibly hazardous things. If feasible, carefully pull your youngster away from harmful items or surfaces.

Time The Seizure: Note the start time of the seizure and note its length. This information will be beneficial for medical personnel in assessing your child's condition.

Protect The Head: If your kid is suffering a generalized tonic-clonic seizure (previously known as grand mal seizure), it is crucial to cushion their head to avoid harm. Place something soft, such as a cushion or folded fabric, beneath their head.

Loosen Tight Clothes: Make sure there are no constrictive articles of clothing, such as ties, scarves, or tight collars, that might obstruct breathing during a seizure. Loosen any restricting clothes around the neck.

Stay At Your Kid's Side: Remain close to your youngster throughout the seizure and give reassurance. Let them know you are available for support and that they are safe.

Clear The Airway: If your kid is unconscious and their breathing gets blocked due to saliva or vomit, gently shift them onto their side to enable the airway to stay open. This may help avoid choking.

Observe And Document: Take note of any particular features during the seizure, such as movements, length, and strange behaviors. This information will be valuable when discussing the experience with healthcare providers.

Time For Recovery: After the seizure finishes, your kid may feel disoriented, puzzled, or fatigued. Give them time to recuperate and restore their composure. Provide a peaceful and encouraging atmosphere.

Seek Medical Treatment: If it's your child's first seizure, lasts more than five minutes, or they have trouble breathing, it's crucial to seek emergency medical attention. Contact emergency services or transport your youngster to the closest hospital.

DON'TS:
Panic Or Restrict Your Kid: It's normal to feel concerned during a seizure but avoid panicking or trying to physically restrain your child. Restraining may possibly injure them or raise the risk of injury.

Insert Items Into The Mouth: Contrary to common perception, you should never put anything in your child's mouth during a seizure. There is no risk of swallowing the tongue, although inserting items may cause damage or restrict the airway.

Try To Wake Them Up Forcefully: Allow the seizure to take its course. Do not try to wake your kid suddenly by shaking or shouting at them. Trying to wake them up abruptly may exacerbate bewilderment and disorientation.

Offer Food Or Drink During A Seizure: Do not try to offer your kid food or water until the seizure has stopped and they are fully aware. During a seizure, swallowing may be difficult and may induce choking.

Provide Medicine (unless prescribed): Unless you have been expressly advised by a healthcare expert to provide medication during a seizure, do not try to do so without adequate instruction.

Neglect Post-seizure Care: After a seizure, it's crucial to offer your kid with a quiet and supportive atmosphere. Do not forget their emotional and physical needs throughout the recuperation phase.

Remember, every child's experience with epilepsy and seizures is unique. It is vital to speak with your child's healthcare physician to build a specific seizure action plan. Educate yourself on epilepsy and seizure management practices to ensure you are well-prepared to face any circumstance that may happen. With correct education and support, you can offer the care your kid needs during a seizure and help them have a full life.

PRACTICAL ISSUES OF CHILDREN LIVING WITH EPILEPSY AND SEIZURES

Living with epilepsy and seizures may bring a number of practical challenges for children and their families. Epilepsy is a neurological illness marked by recurring seizures, and it may have substantial consequences on different elements of a child's life.

While it is essential to highlight that every child's experience with epilepsy is unique, there are certain common practical obstacles that many children with epilepsy endure. These obstacles may impair their daily routine, social interactions, educational possibilities, and general quality of life.

One of the biggest practical challenges encountered by children with epilepsy is the management of their medication. Many children with epilepsy need daily medication to help manage their seizures. However, following medication regimens may be tough, particularly for younger children who may not fully comprehend the need of taking their medicine regularly. This might lead to difficulty in obtaining seizure control and may need regular reminders from parents or caregivers.

Seizures may be unexpected and occur at any moment, which can present safety issues for children with epilepsy. Parents and caregivers need to be careful in maintaining a safe environment for the youngster. They may need to adopt safety precautions such as cushioning sharp edges, fastening furniture, or overseeing activities that might pose a danger during a seizure. Additionally, children with epilepsy may need to be accompanied by an adult while engaging in certain activities, such as swimming or participating in sports, to avoid mishaps or injury during a seizure.

Another practical challenge encountered by children with epilepsy is the possible constraints on their everyday activities. Some children may be advised to avoid specific activities that might induce seizures, such as exposure to flashing lights, severe physical effort, or lack of sleep. These constraints might influence their involvement in leisure activities, sports, or even normal everyday tasks.

Consequently, children with epilepsy may suffer emotions of frustration, loneliness, and a sense of being different from their classmates.

Education is a key element of a child's life, and epilepsy may bring obstacles in this area as well. Seizures may disturb a child's focus and memory, making it difficult for them to keep up with their academics. Frequent absences due to medical visits or recuperation from seizures might also result in lost classroom learning. As a consequence, children with epilepsy may need additional help and accommodations at school, such as extra time for tests, aid with note-taking, or customized assignments to ensure they can fully engage in their education.

Social relationships might be disrupted for children with epilepsy. Due to the unpredictability of seizures, children with epilepsy may feel worried about socializing and engaging in group activities. Fear of having a seizure in public or being ostracized by their peers may lead to social withdrawal, loneliness, and a detrimental influence on self-esteem. Educating students, instructors, and friends about epilepsy may help establish a supportive and inclusive atmosphere.

The emotional well-being of children with epilepsy is also a crucial factor. Living with a chronic disease and suffering recurrent seizures may lead to higher levels of stress, worry, and despair. It is vital for parents, caregivers, and healthcare professionals to offer emotional support, open communication channels, and access to counseling or support groups to assist children to deal with the emotional issues associated with epilepsy.

In conclusion, children living with epilepsy and seizures encounter several practical challenges that might impair their everyday life. Medication management, safety issues, limits on activities, educational obstacles, social interactions, and emotional well-being are all areas that need special attention and assistance. By addressing these practical concerns and providing thorough care, children with epilepsy may have full lives and overcome the obstacles they experience.

MANAGING SEVERE DISABILITIES AND EPILEPSY IN A CHILD

Caring for a kid with severe impairments and epilepsy may be tough, but with the correct knowledge, support, and management measures, parents can help their child experience a full and healthy life. This book seeks to give helpful insights and practical information for parents navigating the complexity of treating chronic disorders. It highlights the significance of providing a supportive environment, developing good communication, maintaining safety, receiving appropriate medical treatment, encouraging social integration, and emphasizing self-care.

Create a Supportive Environment:
It is vital to provide a supporting and caring atmosphere at home. This involves changing the living area to fit the special requirements of your kid, such as incorporating safety measures, ramps, and assistive gadgets. Encourage independence by arranging possessions in an accessible way, and providing adequate room for mobility and rehabilitation activities. Creating a quiet and sensory-friendly atmosphere may also help lessen triggers for seizures.

Establish Effective Communication:
Developing excellent communication methods is vital for both understanding your child's needs and communicating your own concerns. If your kid has limited verbal ability, try alternate ways such as sign language, picture-based communication systems, or assistive technology. Work together with speech therapists and

educators to establish and maintain a consistent communication strategy.

Ensure Safety:
Safety is of essential significance while caring for a kid with severe disability and epilepsy. Take care to limit the chance of accidents or injuries by securing furniture and sharp items, cushioning corners, and keeping a clutter-free environment. In conjunction with medical specialists, prepare a seizure action plan that describes critical procedures during a seizure, including when to provide emergency medicine, if recommended.

Access Appropriate Medical Care:
Establish a close collaboration with healthcare providers that specialize in epilepsy and developmental impairments. Regularly visit with a neurologist competent in treating seizures to check drug efficacy, alter doses, and discuss possible adverse effects. Participate actively at medical visits,

ask questions, and remain informed about new treatment choices or therapies that might help your kid.

Implement Medication Management:
Maintaining an accurate record of your child's medicines, doses, and timetables is vital. Use pill organizers or smartphone applications to organize and monitor prescriptions properly. Be attentive in giving medicines on schedule, and report any changes in your child's condition or adverse effects to the healthcare staff quickly.

Promote Social Integration:
Encourage social contacts and involvement in your child's life. Facilitate chances for your kid to interact with peers via inclusive activities, community initiatives, or special education services. Educate people about your child's illness to develop understanding and acceptance, decreasing the stigma associated with disabilities and epilepsy.

Prioritize Self-Care:
Taking care of a kid with significant disability and epilepsy may be physically and emotionally difficult. It is crucial for parents to emphasize self-care to preserve their own well-being. Seek help from friends, relatives, or support groups that understand the issues you experience. Take pauses when required, explore interests, and dedicate time for relaxation and self-reflection.

Conclusion:
Caring for a kid with significant impairments and epilepsy needs devotion, patience, and a holistic strategy. By creating a supportive environment, establishing effective communication, ensuring safety, accessing appropriate medical care, promoting social integration, and prioritizing self-care, parents can enhance the quality of life for their children while navigating the challenges associated with these conditions. Remember, you are not

alone in this journey, and there are tools and assistance available to help you and your kid flourish.

CHAPTER 2

Challenging Assumptions: Unraveling Misconceptions About Childhood Epilepsy & Seizures

In the world of neurological illnesses, few ailments have managed to engage our interest and create a tapestry of tales quite like epilepsy. An ancient ailment, cloaked in mystery and surrounded by myths, epilepsy has long been enmeshed in a web of mistaken beliefs and changeable superstitions. However, in the ever-evolving landscape of medical knowledge, the moment has come to unravel the riddle that is epilepsy and shed light on its genuine nature.

Welcome to Chapter 2, where we go on a trip through the labyrinth of common myths and discover the firm bedrock of facts about epilepsy and seizures. Here, we shall examine age-old narratives, refute myths that have endured for generations, and replace them with the incontrovertible realities that science has uncovered.

Within these pages, we welcome you to explore a world where seizure activity is frequently misunderstood and misrepresented, leading to the stigmatization and marginalization of people living with epilepsy. Brace yourself as we disentangle the complicated strands of misinformation that have weaved themselves into the fabric of society's view.

We will investigate the depths of the fallacy that all seizures are the same, exposing the remarkable variation within this spectrum of brain occurrences. From the mild absence seizures to the spectacular convulsive episodes, we shall comprehend the astonishing diversity of forms that epilepsy may include.

Prepare to challenge your ideas as we investigate the notion that epilepsy is a curse or a heavenly retribution. We will throw a light on the underlying causes of epilepsy, releasing the load of guilt that has tormented many people throughout history. It is time to replace judgment with empathy, and prejudice with understanding.

As we explore this chapter, we will confront the dangerous myth that epilepsy is infectious, removing the fear and bigotry that have put a shadow across the lives of people afflicted.

No longer will dread and helplessness cloud your actions; instead, you will emerge equipped with the courage to provide assistance and compassion when it counts most.

So, join us as we travel into the depths of human knowledge, exposing the cloud of myths that have hidden the actual nature of epilepsy and seizures. Let us embrace the power of information and tackle the limitations that restrict persons living with epilepsy from having full lives. Together, we will uncover the puzzle, one fact at a time.

MISCONCEPTIONS & FACTS:
MISCONCEPTION: Epilepsy is an uncommon disorder.
FACT: Epilepsy is a reasonably common neurological illness, affecting roughly 1 in 26 individuals at some time in their life.

MISCONCEPTION: All seizures are the same.
FACT: There are several kinds of seizures, including absence seizures, focal seizures, and generalized tonic-clonic seizures, each having distinct symptoms and features.

MISCONCEPTION: Childhood epilepsy is usually caused by brain damage.
FACT: While brain traumas may lead to epilepsy in certain situations, there are

numerous other possible causes, including hereditary factors and unexplained reasons.

MISCONCEPTION: Children with epilepsy are mentally impaired.
FACT: Epilepsy does not inevitably damage a child's IQ. Many children with epilepsy have normal cognitive abilities.

MISCONCEPTION: Epilepsy is communicable.
FACT: Epilepsy is not infectious and cannot be passed from one person to another.

MISCONCEPTION: Children with epilepsy cannot engage in sports or physical activities.
FACT: With good care and supervision, most children with epilepsy may participate in physical activities and sports, although certain restrictions may be required.

MISCONCEPTION: Seizures may be triggered by watching television or using technological gadgets.

FACT: While specific patterns on screens or flashing lights might induce seizures in some persons with photosensitive epilepsy, this is exceedingly uncommon.

MISCONCEPTION: Epilepsy may be healed with an alternative therapy or herbal medicines.

FACT: There is presently no cure for epilepsy. While alternative treatments may help control symptoms in certain circumstances, they should always be used in combination with medical care.

MISCONCEPTION: Febrile convulsions invariably lead to epilepsy.

FACT: Febrile seizures, which occur due to high temperature, are typically innocuous and do not progress to epilepsy in the majority of instances.

MISCONCEPTION: Seizures are usually followed by convulsions or shaking.

FACT: Seizures may manifest in numerous ways, including staring spells, short periods of bewilderment, or transient loss of consciousness without any convulsions.

MISCONCEPTION: All seizures need immediate medical intervention.

FACT: While certain seizures may need urgent medical intervention, many seizures are short and self-resolve without the need for emergency treatment.

MISCONCEPTION: Epilepsy drugs will always create adverse effects.

FACT: While certain epilepsy treatments may have side effects, not all persons will experience them, and the advantages of reducing seizures frequently exceed the possible negative effects.

MISCONCEPTION: Seizures are always provoked by external stimuli.

FACT: Seizures may be induced by several things, including stress, lack of sleep, hormonal changes, or certain drugs, but they can also occur spontaneously without any recognized trigger.

MISCONCEPTION: Children with epilepsy should be handled differently or isolated from social activities.
FACT: Children with epilepsy should be treated like any other kid and encouraged to engage in social activities. Educating people about epilepsy may help create an inclusive atmosphere.

MISCONCEPTION: Epilepsy is usually a lifetime affliction.
FACT: While epilepsy is a lifelong disorder for many people, some children may outgrow their seizures as they mature.

MISCONCEPTION: Children with epilepsy have an increased risk of sudden unexplained death.

FACT: While sudden unexplained death in epilepsy (SUDEP) is a worry, it is quite uncommon, and most children with epilepsy do not have an elevated risk of this occurring.

MISCONCEPTION: Seizures are usually preceded by an aura or warning symptoms.
FACT: While some seizures may be preceded by an aura or warning symptoms, many occur without any previous indication.

MISCONCEPTION: Epilepsy solely impacts physical health.
FACT: Epilepsy may have numerous implications on a child's life, including emotional, social, and scholastic elements. Support from healthcare experts, teachers, and peers is vital.

MISCONCEPTION: It's preferable to restrain or hold a youngster during a seizure.

FACT: During a seizure, it is crucial to safeguard the child's safety by eliminating any close items that may cause injury. However, it is not advisable to restrain or hold them down.

MISCONCEPTION: Seizures are usually painful for the youngster.
FACT: Seizures themselves are not often painful for the youngster. However, injuries acquired during a seizure, such as biting the tongue or falling, might cause discomfort.

MISCONCEPTION: Epilepsy is a consequence of bad parenting or psychological disorders.
FACT: Epilepsy is a neurological illness and is not caused by parenting style or psychological factors.

MISCONCEPTION: Children with epilepsy should avoid swimming or bathing.
FACT: With sufficient measures, such as monitoring and perhaps utilizing life

jackets, most children with epilepsy may safely engage in swimming or bathing activities.

MISCONCEPTION: Epilepsy is an impediment to academic achievement.
FACT: With adequate care and assistance, most children with epilepsy can excel academically and attain their full potential.

MISCONCEPTION: All seizures are life-threatening situations.
FACT: While certain seizures may be medical crises, most seizures are not life-threatening, and generally recover spontaneously.

MISCONCEPTION: Children with epilepsy are more prone to mood problems.
FACT: Children with epilepsy may have a slightly greater chance of developing mood disorders such as depression or anxiety, however not all people will suffer these illnesses.

MISCONCEPTION: Epilepsy may be induced by vaccines.

FACT: Extensive study has proven no relationship between immunizations and the development of epilepsy or seizures.

MISCONCEPTION: A person may swallow their tongue during a seizure.

FACT: It is not feasible for a person to swallow their tongue during a seizure. Trying to put anything in their mouth may possibly do damage.

MISCONCEPTION: Seizures invariably end in loss of consciousness.

FACT: While certain seizures may induce loss of consciousness, many seizures do not, and the sufferer may remain aware of their surroundings.

MISCONCEPTION: Children with epilepsy should avoid participating in school field excursions.

FACT: With good preparation and communication between parents, teachers, and healthcare experts, children with epilepsy may safely participate in school field excursions.

MISCONCEPTION: Epilepsy is a progressive condition.
FACT: Epilepsy itself is not a progressive condition, although the frequency or severity of seizures might fluctuate with time in certain people.

MISCONCEPTION: Epilepsy may be healed by surgery.
FACT: Surgery may be an option for some persons with epilepsy, but it is not a sure cure, and not all individuals are candidates for surgical intervention.

MISCONCEPTION: All children with epilepsy need special education assistance.
FACT: While some children with epilepsy may need more educational assistance, not

all children will need special education
programs.

MISCONCEPTION: Seizures may be
avoided by avoiding strong lights or
particular meals.
FACT: While photosensitive epilepsy may
be caused by particular light patterns,
avoiding bright lights or certain meals will
not prevent seizures in most instances.

MISCONCEPTION: Epilepsy is a
consequence of supernatural or spiritual
forces.
FACT: Epilepsy is a medical disorder with
recognized neurological origins and is not
induced by supernatural or spiritual forces.

MISCONCEPTION: Children with
epilepsy should never take part in
sleepovers or overnight activities.
FACT: With sufficient preparation and
communication, children with epilepsy may
participate in sleepovers and overnight

events, assuring their safety and enough supervision.

MISCONCEPTION: Epilepsy is a symptom of inferior intellect.
FACT: Epilepsy has no clear association with IQ. Many children with epilepsy have normal or above-average IQ.

MISCONCEPTION: All seizures need medical care.
FACT: Some seizures may not need urgent medical attention, particularly if they are short and the kid has a known epilepsy diagnosis. However, it is vital to speak with a healthcare practitioner for thorough assessment and counseling.

MISCONCEPTION: Epilepsy drugs usually lead to weight gain.
FACT: While weight gain may be a side effect of certain epilepsy treatments, not all persons will experience this, and it can vary from person to person.

MISCONCEPTION: It's preferable to keep epilepsy a secret to prevent stigma.

FACT: Open communication and education about epilepsy may help eliminate stigma and establish a supportive environment for the kid. It is crucial to educate people about epilepsy to encourage understanding.

MISCONCEPTION: Children with epilepsy should avoid stress or excitement.

FACT: While stress or excitement might possibly provoke seizures in certain people, it is not essential to totally avoid these feelings. Managing stress and establishing coping techniques might be useful.

MISCONCEPTION: Epilepsy primarily affects younger children.

FACT: Epilepsy may affect persons of all ages, including teenagers and adults.

MISCONCEPTION: A single seizure always implies epilepsy.

FACT: A single seizure does not always signify a person has epilepsy. Epilepsy is generally diagnosed when a person suffers recurring seizures over time.

MISCONCEPTION: Children with epilepsy should never take baths.
FACT: With adequate supervision and safeguards, such as using a non-slip mat, children with epilepsy may safely take baths.

MISCONCEPTION: Children with epilepsy cannot have a normal life.
FACT: With adequate management, therapy, and support, most children with epilepsy may enjoy a full and active life, engaging in many activities and reaching their objectives.

MISCONCEPTION: All seizures need contacting an ambulance.
FACT: While certain seizures may need emergency medical assistance, not all seizures demand calling an ambulance.

Knowing the child's seizure treatment strategy may assist establish the right reaction.

MISCONCEPTION: Children with epilepsy cannot have pets.
FACT: With adequate supervision and safety precautions, children with epilepsy can have pets. Pets may give companionship and emotional support.

MISCONCEPTION: Epilepsy is an indication of a mental disorder.
FACT: Epilepsy is a neurological ailment and is not directly related with mental illness. However, persons with epilepsy may have an increased risk of acquiring certain mental health issues.

MISCONCEPTION: Children with epilepsy should avoid engaging in physical education sessions.
FACT: With adequate monitoring and communication between parents,

instructors, and healthcare experts, most children with epilepsy may safely participate in physical education programs.

MISCONCEPTION: Epilepsy is usually obvious and immediately detectable.
FACT: Epilepsy is not always obvious, and some persons may have seizures that are not easily evident to others. It is crucial to be aware of varied seizure presentations.

MISCONCEPTION: Seizures may be halted by restraining or holding the victim down.
FACT: Restraining or holding down a person during a seizure might possibly cause injury and is not advised. It is preferable to safeguard their safety by eliminating adjacent items and creating a safe atmosphere.

MISCONCEPTION: Children with epilepsy are restricted in professional opportunities.

FACT: With adequate treatment and control of seizures, most children with epilepsy may pursue a broad variety of professional opportunities. The professional selection should be based on individual strengths and interests.

MISCONCEPTION: Seizures are usually preceded by a smell or taste sensation.
FACT: While certain seizures may be followed by olfactory or gustatory sensations, not all seizures have these prior symptoms.

MISCONCEPTION: Epilepsy is usually a permanent disability.
FACT: While epilepsy is a chronic disorder for many people, some children may outgrow their seizures with age and may no longer need therapy or have seizures.

CHAPTER 3

Unveiling the Hidden Avenues: Nurturing Hope through Complementary and Alternative Treatments

In the arena of juvenile epilepsy, a diagnosis frequently thrusts families into a world of uncertainty, where every seizure contains a plethora of questions and anxieties. Traditional drugs and treatments clearly play a significant part in controlling this neurological illness, but there exists a wide tapestry of untapped options that may give fresh rays of hope. Welcome to a chapter that uncovers the secret channels of complementary and alternative therapies, where ancient knowledge dances with current science to highlight potential approaches for seizure control and enhanced quality of life for children with epilepsy.

In this chapter, we begin on a thrilling examination of unusual treatment approaches, diving into the domain of complementary and alternative medicine (CAM).

Often brushed aside by conventional medical discourse, CAM throws a spotlight on therapeutic techniques that complement established therapies or stand alone as alternative possibilities. From natural cures rooted in centuries-old knowledge to innovative therapies leveraging the power of technology, we go across the wide terrain of treatments that sit outside the standard medical paradigm.

As we travel this intriguing landscape, we find an assortment of techniques that include mind, body, and spirit. We discover traditional techniques such as acupuncture, which provide distinct insights on restoring balance and fostering general well-being. We meet novel treatments, such as biofeedback, which try to harness the brain's intrinsic capacity to self-regulate. And we discover the knowledge of herbal treatments and vitamins, handed down through centuries, bringing glimpses of alleviation and control.

However, before proceeding further, it is vital to examine this chapter with a careful eye. We investigate these alternate options not as a rejection of conventional medical procedures, but as an encouragement to extend our knowledge and adopt a more holistic approach to epilepsy care. It is an invitation to investigate the possible synergies that may exist between conventional and alternative therapies, picturing a future where individualized, integrated care becomes the standard.

So, my reader, join us on this informative adventure as we discover the untapped potential of complementary and alternative therapy for epilepsy and seizures in children. Together, let us open our minds to the endless possibilities that lie inside, motivated by the promise of empowering families and paving the road toward a better future for individuals living with epilepsy.

INTRODUCTION TO COMPLEMENTARY AND ALTERNATIVE TREATMENTS
- Understanding the notion of complementary and alternative therapies
- Their role in controlling epilepsy and seizures

In recent years, there has been a rising interest in complementary and alternative therapies for many health concerns, especially those affecting children. Complementary and alternative medicine (CAM) comprises a broad variety of treatments and practices that are not normally considered part of standard Western medicine. Instead, CAM methods strive to offer comprehensive treatment by concentrating on the physical, mental, and emotional well-being of people. This article will offer an introduction to the notion of complementary and alternative therapies for kids, with a special emphasis on their function in controlling epilepsy and seizures in children.

UNDERSTANDING THE CONCEPT OF COMPLEMENTARY AND ALTERNATIVE TREATMENTS

Complementary and alternative treatments are commonly utilized alongside traditional medical therapy to boost general health and well-being. These therapies may include herbal medicines, nutritional supplements, mind-body practices, acupuncture, chiropractic care, massage therapy, and many more. The main premise of CAM is to assist the body's inherent healing mechanisms and create balance and harmony.

When it comes to children, complementary and alternative therapies may provide a non-invasive and drug-free approach to addressing numerous health concerns. They are typically viewed as a more gentle and natural manner of promoting a child's health and development. However, it is vital to highlight that not all CAM treatments have been fully investigated or proved beneficial, and their usage should always be reviewed with healthcare experts.

THEIR ROLE IN MANAGING EPILEPSY AND SEIZURES

While conventional medical treatments, such as anti-seizure medications, are the primary approach to managing epilepsy, complementary and alternative treatments can play a supportive role in reducing seizure frequency, improving overall well-being, and enhancing the effectiveness of conventional therapies.

One regularly utilized CAM treatment for epilepsy is food therapy. The ketogenic diet, for example, is a high-fat, low-carbohydrate diet that has shown encouraging effects in lowering seizures, especially in children with epilepsy that does not react well to medication. The diet works by generating a condition of ketosis in the body, which affects the metabolism of the brain and lowers seizure activity.

In addition to food treatment, various CAM techniques such as acupuncture, yoga, and biofeedback have been examined in controlling epilepsy in children. Acupuncture, a method originating from Traditional Chinese Medicine, involves the insertion of tiny needles into particular sites on the body to enhance energy flow and create balance. Some research shows that acupuncture may help lessen the frequency and severity of seizures in children with epilepsy.

Yoga, a mind-body practice that incorporates physical postures, breathing exercises, and meditation, has also shown potential in controlling epilepsy. It may help relieve tension, induce relaxation, and enhance general well-being. While the evidence supporting yoga's usefulness in epilepsy therapy is currently limited, several studies have revealed excellent effects in terms of seizure control and quality of life in children.

Biofeedback is another CAM treatment that may be effective for children with epilepsy. It includes teaching people to manage their physiological processes, such as heart rate, blood pressure, and brainwave activity, using input from monitoring equipment. By learning to manage these processes, children may be able to minimize seizure activity and enhance their general functioning.

It is vital to underline that complementary and alternative therapies should always be used in combination with standard medical therapy for epilepsy. Parents and caregivers should engage together with healthcare experts to ensure the safe and successful integration of CAM treatments into a complete treatment plan for their child.

CONCLUSION
Complementary and alternative therapies may give essential help in treating numerous health disorders in children, including epilepsy. While these treatments should never replace traditional medical care, they may be used in concert with it to increase general well-being and perhaps lessen the frequency and severity of seizures.

However, it is vital to approach CAM therapies with caution, contact healthcare specialists, and confirm that the selected treatments are safe and suitable for the child's unique situation. By adopting an integrated approach, parents and caregivers may offer holistic care for their children, increasing their health and quality of life.

DIET AND NUTRITION
- The ketogenic diet and its influence on epilepsy
- Other dietary options for treating seizures
- Nutritional concerns for children with epilepsy

Complementary and alternative therapies, including food and nutrition, play a key role in controlling numerous health disorders in children. In the case of epilepsy and seizures, numerous dietary methods have shown promise in lowering seizure frequency and enhancing general well-being. Two common dietary therapies for epilepsy include the ketogenic diet and various dietary regimens, both of which need careful nutritional considerations.

THE KETOGENIC DIET AND ITS IMPACT ON EPILEPSY

The ketogenic diet is a high-fat, low-carbohydrate, and adequate-protein diet that has been used for over a century to control epilepsy, particularly in children who do not respond to typical antiepileptic drugs. The diet's main purpose is to produce a state of ketosis in the body when ketones generated from fats become the predominant fuel supply for the brain instead of glucose.

The ketogenic diet is commonly given under medical supervision since it needs stringent adherence and monitoring. It often consists of a ratio of fats to carbs and proteins, such as 4:1 or 3:1. This indicates that for every gram of carbs and proteins, four or three grams of fats are ingested, respectively. The diet is highly personalized and suited to each child's exact requirements, taking into consideration their age, weight, and activity level.

The influence of the ketogenic diet on children with epilepsy may be profound. The high-fat content of the diet changes the metabolism, resulting in ketosis. Ketones are considered to have antiepileptic properties, helping to lessen seizure frequency and severity. Additionally, the ketogenic diet may have additional good impacts, including better cognitive performance, greater alertness, and enhanced general well-being in certain youngsters.

OTHER DIETARY APPROACHES FOR MANAGING SEIZURES:
In addition to the ketogenic diet, numerous additional dietary methods have shown promise in controlling seizures in children. These options may be explored as alternatives when the ketogenic diet is not suited or preferred:

a. Modified Atkins Diet (MAD): The modified Atkins diet is a less stringent variation of the ketogenic diet that permits somewhat more carbs and protein consumption while still encouraging a state of ketosis. It may be more tolerable for certain children and their families while still delivering possible seizure control.

b. Low Glycemic Index Treatment (LGIT): The LGIT focuses on ingesting meals with a low glycemic index, meaning they promote a slower and more steady increase in blood sugar levels. This strategy seeks to normalize blood glucose levels and may help decrease seizure frequency.

c. Medium-Chain Triglyceride (MCT) Ketogenic Diet: This diet contains a larger consumption of medium-chain triglycerides, which are rapidly turned into ketones by the liver. It allows for a little increased carbohydrate consumption while still producing ketosis.

d. Modified Fasting: Periodic fasting or modified fasting includes reducing calorie consumption for a specified time, followed by a regular diet. This method may have good benefits on seizure management, however, it needs careful monitoring and medical supervision.

NUTRITIONAL CONSIDERATIONS FOR CHILDREN WITH EPILEPSY:
When adopting any dietary intervention for controlling epilepsy in children, various nutritional concerns should be taken into account:

a. Adequate Nutrient Intake: Since the ketogenic diet and other dietary methods limit some food categories, great attention must be made to ensure children acquire all critical nutrients. Nutritional supplements or specialized meal choices may be essential to suit their demands.

b. Fluid and Electrolyte Balance: Diets like the ketogenic diet might raise the risk of dehydration and electrolyte abnormalities. Sufficient fluid intake and suitable electrolyte supplements may be important, particularly during the early adaption period.

c. Growth and Development: Children have specific dietary needs for growth and development. Regular monitoring of growth markers, including weight and height, is necessary to ensure that dietary changes do not impair their nutritional status.

d. Regular Monitoring and Evaluation: Regular medical and nutritional monitoring are needed for children following a customized diet for epilepsy. This involves periodic check-ups, blood tests, and evaluation of seizure control, as well as monitoring for any possible side effects or nutritional deficiencies.

In conclusion, complementary and alternative therapies, including dietary interventions, offer useful choices for controlling epilepsy and seizures in children. The ketogenic diet and other dietary therapies, when adopted under medical supervision, may greatly enhance seizure management and improve the general well-being of children with epilepsy. However, it is vital to consider individual nutritional demands and regularly evaluate the child's health during the dietary intervention.

HERBAL REMEDIES AND SUPPLEMENTS

- **Exploring herbal medicines and their potential benefits**
- **Commonly used supplements for epilepsy treatment**
- **Safety considerations and precautions**

While traditional medical therapies such as antiepileptic medicines (AEDs) are regularly provided to control epilepsy, some parents may explore other options, including herbal remedies and supplements, to complement their child's therapy. It's crucial to remember that herbal medicines and supplements should always be taken under the advice of a healthcare practitioner, and their efficacy may differ for each person. Here, we'll review various herbal medicines and supplements that are regularly used and highlight safety issues and warnings for children with epilepsy and seizures.

HERBAL REMEDIES FOR CHILDREN WITH EPILEPSY AND SEIZURES:

CBD (Cannabidiol): CBD is a chemical produced from the cannabis plant that has attracted interest for its possible anticonvulsant qualities. It has been researched for its efficacy in lowering seizure frequency in some kinds of epilepsy, including Dravet syndrome and

Lennox-Gastaut syndrome. However, the use of CBD for children with epilepsy should be done under medical supervision, since it may interact with other drugs and may have negative effects.

Passionflower (Passiflora incarnata): Passionflower is a herb recognized for its soothing qualities and has been historically used to address anxiety and sleep difficulties. Some studies show that passionflower may have anticonvulsant qualities, but further study is required to verify its effectiveness and safety in children with epilepsy.

Valerian (Valeriana officinalis): Valerian is a plant often used for its sedative and relaxing qualities. While it is usually used to help sleep, some anecdotal accounts indicate that valerian may potentially have antiepileptic properties. However, more scientific research are necessary to substantiate these claims and identify acceptable doses for youngsters.

Bacopa (Bacopa monnieri): Bacopa is a herb widely used in Ayurvedic medicine to boost cognitive function and memory. It includes active chemicals that may have neuroprotective benefits and perhaps lessen seizure activity. However, comprehensive clinical studies are required to validate its safety and effectiveness in children with cpilepsy.

SUPPLEMENTS FOR EPILEPSY MANAGEMENT IN CHILDREN:
Vitamin B6 (Pyridoxine): Vitamin B6 is involved in several metabolic activities in the body, including neurotransmitter production. Some studies show that supplementation with vitamin B6 may help decrease seizures in children with specific kinds of epilepsy, such as pyridoxine-dependent epilepsy. However, it is vital to speak with a healthcare

practitioner to identify proper doses and monitor any adverse effects.

Magnesium: Magnesium is a vital mineral involved in numerous physiological activities, including nerve transmission and muscle relaxation. Some studies have suggested that magnesium supplementation may have a favorable impact on seizure management, especially in children with magnesium shortage or specific kinds of epilepsy. Again, competent medical assistance is important to identify the ideal dose and monitor magnesium levels.

SAFETY CONCERNS AND PRECAUTIONS FOR CHILDREN WITH EPILEPSY AND SEIZURES:
Always Contact A Healthcare Expert: It is vital to include a healthcare professional, ideally a pediatric neurologist or epileptologist, in the treatment of epilepsy and the use of herbal therapies and supplements. They can give accurate

diagnoses, advise suitable treatment approaches, and assure the safety and well-being of the kid.

Be Careful Of Possible Interactions: Herbal remedies and supplements may interact with prescription drugs used to control epilepsy, possibly lowering their efficacy or producing bad effects. It is crucial to notify the healthcare practitioner about any herbs or supplements being taken to avoid such interactions.

Quality And Standardization: When contemplating herbal medicines or supplements, seek renowned companies that conform to quality standards and have completed third-party testing. This assures that the items are free from contaminants and appropriately labeled on their ingredients and strength.

Individual Variations And Monitoring: Every kid with epilepsy is unique, and what works for one may not work for another. It is vital to thoroughly evaluate the child's reaction to any herbal therapies or supplements and make modifications as required under physician supervision.

Never quit prescription medication: Herbal treatments and supplements should not be used as a replacement for approved antiepileptic medicines. It is vital to maintain the recommended pharmaceutical regimen unless expressly advised by a healthcare expert.

In summary, although herbal medicines and supplements may have potential advantages for children with epilepsy and seizures, they should always be taken under the advice of a healthcare practitioner. Proper medical supervision guarantees the safety and proper use of these therapies, alongside traditional treatments, in treating epilepsy and maximizing the child's well-being.

MIND-BODY TECHNIQUES

- Introduction to mind-body techniques for epilepsy
- Stress management and relaxation approaches
- Biofeedback and neurofeedback

Mind-body methods are holistic approaches that concentrate on the connectivity of the mind, body, and emotions to enhance total well-being. These strategies have demonstrated promising outcomes in addressing numerous health issues, including epilepsy and seizures in children. While medicine and medical treatments remain vital in the treatment of epilepsy, mind-body activities may complement conventional therapies by lowering stress, encouraging relaxation, and improving the general quality of life.

STRESS MANAGEMENT AND RELAXATION TECHNIQUES FOR KIDS WITH EPILEPSY AND SEIZURES:
Stress is a recognized cause of seizures in patients with epilepsy. Therefore, teaching stress management and relaxation strategies to children with epilepsy may help lessen the frequency and severity of seizures. Here are some good techniques:

Deep Breathing: Deep breathing activities, such as diaphragmatic breathing, may stimulate the body's relaxation response. Encourage youngsters to take calm, deep breaths, filling their lungs completely and expelling gently.

Progressive Muscle Relaxation: This method includes tensing and releasing various muscle groups to produce relaxation. Children may be directed through a series of muscle groups, helping them learn to detect and release tension.

Guided Imagery: Guided imagery is employing visualizations to create a quiet and pleasant mental state. Children may be led to picture calm sceneries or use their senses to imagine relaxing experiences.

Mindfulness Meditation: Mindfulness meditation encourages children to be present in the now, observing their thoughts and feelings without judgment. It may help relieve stress and promote emotional well-being.

Yoga and Tai Chi: These mild movement activities combine breath control, stretching, and relaxation methods. They may boost physical flexibility, decrease tension, and foster a feeling of calm in children with epilepsy.

BIOFEEDBACK AND NEUROFEEDBACK FOR KIDS WITH EPILEPSY AND SEIZURES:

Biofeedback and neurofeedback approaches try to educate people on how to manage their physiological reactions, such as heart rate, muscular tension, and brainwave patterns. These approaches may be effective for children with epilepsy in the following ways:

Biofeedback: Biofeedback includes employing electrical sensors to monitor physiological processes in real time. Children may learn to notice and manage their body's reactions. For instance, people may utilize biofeedback to learn how to minimize muscular tension or control their heart rate, possibly lowering seizure triggers.

Neurofeedback: Neurofeedback focuses on educating people to manage their brainwave activity. Children with epilepsy may learn to self-regulate their brainwave patterns, supporting enhanced brain function and perhaps lowering the incidence of seizures.

Both biofeedback and neurofeedback need the direction of qualified specialists who can offer feedback and assist youngsters develop self-regulation abilities.

Conclusion:
Mind-body approaches provide intriguing prospects for children with epilepsy and seizures. Stress management and relaxation practices may help children lower stress levels and generate a feeling of calm, thereby decreasing seizure triggers. Biofeedback and neurofeedback approaches allow children to detect and manage their physiological reactions, leading to greater seizure control. However, it is vital to emphasize that mind-body therapies should be utilized as complementary approaches alongside established medical treatments, and collaboration with healthcare specialists is necessary for a thorough treatment plan for children with epilepsy and seizures.

ACUPUNCTURE AND ACUPRESSURE

- Understanding acupuncture and its possible effects on seizures
- Acupressure as a supplementary treatment for controlling epilepsy
- Seeking a competent practitioner

Acupuncture and acupressure are alternative treatments that have been utilized for generations in traditional Chinese medicine. While the main therapy for epilepsy in children includes medication and other medical treatments, some parents and caregivers may investigate alternative therapies like acupuncture and acupressure to control seizures and enhance overall well-being.

In this part, we will go into understanding acupuncture and acupressure, their possible benefits on seizures for kids with epilepsy, and how to identify a trained practitioner for these therapies.

UNDERSTANDING ACUPUNCTURE AND ITS POTENTIAL EFFECTS ON SEIZURES FOR KIDS:

Acupuncture is the insertion of tiny needles into particular spots on the body. According to traditional Chinese medicine, these points relate to energy routes or meridians that may be activated to restore balance and promote healing. The purpose of acupuncture is to increase the flow of energy, known as Qi, throughout the body.

When it comes to epilepsy in children, acupuncture is regarded to possibly aid by:

a) Reducing Seizure Frequency: Some research shows that acupuncture may help lessen the frequency and severity of seizures in children with epilepsy. It is thought that acupuncture induces the production of endorphins and neurotransmitters that have a relaxing impact on the nervous system.

b) Improving Overall Well-being: Children with epilepsy may endure physical and mental stress. Acupuncture is renowned for its ability to induce relaxation, decrease anxiety, and enhance sleep quality. By addressing these factors, acupuncture may indirectly assist in a better treatment of seizures.

ACUPRESSURE AS A COMPLEMENTARY THERAPY FOR MANAGING EPILEPSY IN CHILDREN:

Acupressure is a method similar to acupuncture, except instead of using needles, pressure is delivered to particular areas of the body. This pressure may be provided by light massage, finger pressure, or even utilizing tiny devices developed for acupressure.

For children with epilepsy, acupressure may give the following possible benefits:

a) Calming the Nervous System: Acupressure treatments given to particular areas may assist trigger the body's relaxation response, decreasing tension and anxiety levels in children with epilepsy.

b) Supporting Overall Well-being: Acupressure may promote better sleep, decrease muscular tension, and boost overall well-being. By offering a sensation of ease and relaxation, acupressure may indirectly benefit seizure control.

It's crucial to remember that although some patients may experience beneficial outcomes from acupuncture and acupressure, these treatments should always be used as complementary to medical care and not as a substitute for prescription medicine or other interventions.

SEEKING A QUALIFIED PRACTITIONER OF ACUPUNCTURE AND ACUPRESSURE FOR THE TREATMENT OF EPILEPSY AND SEIZURES IN KIDS:
When contemplating acupuncture or acupressure for a kid with epilepsy, it is vital

to identify a skilled practitioner with expertise in treating pediatric patients. Here are some methods to aid you with your search:

a) Research and Referrals: Start by researching reputable acupuncture and acupressure practitioners in your region. Seek referrals from healthcare specialists, such as pediatricians or neurologists, who may have information on practitioners specialized in epilepsy.

b) Credentials and Training: Look for practitioners who are licensed or qualified in acupuncture or acupressure. They should have undergone sufficient training and have expertise in treating children with epilepsy or seizure disorders.

b) Consultation and Evaluation: Schedule a consultation with the practitioner to review your child's individual requirements and medical history. The practitioner should be attentive, ask pertinent questions, and offer clear explanations of how acupuncture or acupressure may assist your kid.

d) contact with the Medical Team: It is crucial to maintain open contact between the acupuncture/acupressure practitioner and your child's medical team. This promotes a coordinated approach and enables information exchange that may aid in enhancing the overall care and treatment of your child's epilepsy.

e) Monitoring and Evaluation: Keep note of your child's improvement during acupuncture or acupressure treatments. Note any changes in seizure frequency, severity, or general well-being. Share this information with both the practitioner and the medical team to assess the success of the therapy.

Remember, the safety and well-being of your kid should always be the main concern.

Before initiating any complementary treatment, contact your child's healthcare physician to confirm it is suitable and safe for your child's individual condition.

In summary, acupuncture and acupressure may provide potential advantages as supplementary therapy for children with epilepsy. They have the potential to help regulate seizures, decrease stress and anxiety, and enhance general well-being. However, it is vital to speak with trained practitioners knowledgeable in treating young children with epilepsy and maintain contact with your child's medical team throughout the process.

CHIROPRACTIC CARE
- Chiropractic therapy for epilepsy and seizures
- Assessing the safety and effectiveness of chiropractic care
- Integrating chiropractic care into an overall treatment plan

Chiropractic treatment is a comprehensive approach to healthcare that focuses on the musculoskeletal system, especially the spine, and its influence on general health and well-being. While chiropractic treatment is generally linked with treating problems such as back pain, it has also been examined as a viable supplemental therapy for epilepsy and seizures in children.

In this part, we will review chiropractic therapy for epilepsy and seizures in children, analyze the safety and effectiveness of chiropractic care in kids, and investigate the integration of chiropractic care into an overall treatment plan for children with epilepsy.

CHIROPRACTIC TREATMENT FOR EPILEPSY AND SEIZURES IN CHILDREN: Chiropractic therapy for epilepsy and seizures in children attempts to increase the body's inherent healing mechanisms and promote normal neurological function. Chiropractors think that misalignments called subluxations in the spine may interrupt the regular flow of nerve impulses and influence the entire functioning of the body, including the brain. By applying manual adjustment procedures, chiropractors try to rectify these subluxations and restore appropriate nerve function, possibly decreasing seizure activity in children.

Chiropractic therapy for children with epilepsy often requires a full review of the child's medical history, physical examination, and sometimes diagnostic imaging. Chiropractors may utilize a range of treatments, including spine adjustments, joint mobility, soft tissue manipulation, and lifestyle counseling to address the underlying conditions leading to seizures. The treatment approach is personalized depending on the child's particular requirements and may entail recurring sessions over a period of time.

ASSESSING THE SAFETY AND EFFICACY OF CHIROPRACTIC CARE IN KIDS:
When contemplating chiropractic therapy for children, safety is of fundamental significance. Chiropractors who specialize in pediatric treatment have additional training and a strong awareness of the unique requirements and concerns of young patients. They apply gentle, age-appropriate procedures and customize the therapy to guarantee the comfort and safety of the kid.

While there is minimal scientific study explicitly evaluating the efficacy of chiropractic therapy for epilepsy and seizures in children, some anecdotal data shows that chiropractic treatment may have a favorable influence. However, it is crucial to stress that chiropractic therapy should not be considered as a replacement for standard medical care or anti-seizure medicines. It should be seen as a supplemental treatment that may bring extra support and advantages.

INTEGRATING CHIROPRACTIC CARE INTO AN OVERALL TREATMENT PLAN IN KIDS:
When contemplating chiropractic therapy for children with epilepsy, it is vital to have open communication and cooperation amongst the child's healthcare professionals. Chiropractors should work in concert with the child's physician, neurologist, and other professionals engaged in their care to establish a thorough and coherent treatment plan.

Integrating chiropractic therapy into an entire treatment plan may require frequent contact between the multiple healthcare professionals, exchange of medical information and test findings, and cooperative decision-making about the child's treatment choices. This collaborative approach helps ensure that all elements of the child's health are evaluated, and any possible contraindications or interactions are discovered.

It is also crucial for parents or guardians to be actively engaged in their child's care and to speak freely with the healthcare staff. They should notify all clinicians about any chiropractic treatments their kid is getting, as well as any changes or improvements they detect in their child's seizure activity.

In conclusion, chiropractic therapy for epilepsy and seizures in children strives to maximize neurological function by treating subluxations in the spine.
While greater study is required to show the effectiveness of chiropractic care for juvenile epilepsy, it may function as a complementary therapy that, when incorporated into an overall treatment plan, might possibly give extra support for children with seizures.

It is crucial for parents and healthcare practitioners to work together to guarantee the safety and well-being of the kid and to make educated choices about their care.

TRADITIONAL CHINESE MEDICINE (TCM)
- Introduction to TCM and its holistic approach
- Herbal medication and acupuncture in TCM for epilepsy
- Working with a TCM practitioner

Traditional Chinese Medicine (TCM) is an ancient medicinal system that has been practiced for thousands of years in China and other areas of East Asia. It is founded on the notion that the body and mind are interrelated, and strives to restore balance and harmony within the body to promote health and well-being. TCM offers a holistic approach to treatment, evaluating not just the physical symptoms but also the underlying imbalances and the individual's whole constitution.

When it comes to the treatment of epilepsy and seizures in children, TCM provides a unique viewpoint and a spectrum of therapeutic techniques. TCM sees epilepsy as a consequence of imbalances in the body's essential energy, known as Qi, as well as disturbances in the movement of blood and other biological components. The purpose of TCM therapy for epilepsy in children is to control and harmonize these imbalances, hence minimizing the frequency and severity of seizures.

HERBAL MEDICINE AND ACUPUNCTURE IN TCM FOR EPILEPSY AND SEIZURES IN KIDS:
One of the basic therapy techniques in TCM is herbal medicine. TCM practitioners prescribe a mixture of herbs that are thought to have unique qualities to correct

the imbalances linked with epilepsy in children. These herbal formulas are often personalized to each individual's particular condition and may comprise a range of substances such as roots, leaves, bark, and minerals. The precise herbs used and their combinations are decided by the TCM practitioner depending on the child's symptoms, constitution, and underlying pattern of imbalance.

Acupuncture is another key component of TCM for treating epilepsy and seizures in youngsters. Acupuncture includes the insertion of fine needles into certain sites on the body, which are thought to alter the flow of Qi and restore equilibrium. In the case of epilepsy, acupuncture points may be targeted to treat the precise imbalances causing seizures. Acupuncture may assist regulate the nervous system, induce relaxation, and enhance general well-being.

WORKING WITH A TCM PRACTITIONER FOR EPILEPSY AND SEIZURES IN KIDS:

If you are contemplating TCM for your child's epilepsy or seizures, it is crucial to work with a skilled and experienced TCM practitioner. Here are some crucial processes involved in engaging with a TCM practitioner:

Initial examination: The TCM practitioner will do a complete examination of your child's medical history, symptoms, and general health. They may inquire about the frequency and type of seizures, any triggers, and any other pertinent information. The practitioner will also monitor the child's tongue, pulse, and other bodily indications to discover the underlying pattern of imbalance.

Treatment Plan: Based on the evaluation, the TCM practitioner will build a tailored treatment plan for your kid. This plan may include herbal medication, acupuncture, nutritional suggestions, lifestyle adjustments, and other TCM treatments as considered suitable.

Herbal Medicine Prescription: The TCM practitioner will prescribe a special herbal composition customized to your child's condition. The herbs may be administered in the form of teas, powders, capsules, or tablets. It is vital to follow the suggested dose and advise the practitioner about any changes or improvements in your child's health.

Acupuncture Appointments: If acupuncture is part of the treatment plan, the TCM practitioner will arrange frequent acupuncture appointments for your kid. During the sessions, the practitioner will implant small needles into particular acupuncture sites, often keeping them in place for a brief length of time. The amount and frequency of acupuncture treatments will depend on the particular requirements of the kid.

Follow-up And Monitoring: Regular follow-up appointments will be planned to evaluate your child's development and make any required modifications to the treatment plan. It is vital to speak honestly with the TCM practitioner and offer feedback on your child's symptoms, particularly any changes in seizure frequency or severity.

It is vital to emphasize that TCM should not be used as a substitute for standard medical therapy for epilepsy. TCM may be utilized as a supplementary therapy alongside conventional treatment, with good cooperation between the TCM practitioner and the child's main healthcare provider.

Conclusion:
Traditional Chinese Medicine (TCM) provides a comprehensive approach to the treatment of epilepsy and seizures in

children. Through the use of herbal medicine, acupuncture, and other TCM methods, TCM practitioners strive to restore balance and harmony within the body, therefore lowering the frequency and severity of seizures. Working with a trained TCM practitioner may assist build a specific treatment plan for your kid, addressing their individual requirements and imbalances. However, it is crucial to combine TCM with conventional medical treatment and to maintain open communication between the TCM practitioner and the child's healthcare team.

AYURVEDA
- Understanding the Ayurvedic method of medicine
- Ayurvedic herbs and remedies for epilepsy management
- Combining Ayurveda with mainstream epilepsy therapies

Ayurveda is an ancient system of medicine that began in India thousands of years ago. It emphasizes on establishing balance and harmony in the body, mind, and spirit to improve total health and well-being. Ayurveda tackles health and healing from a holistic viewpoint and provides a variety of medicines, therapies, and lifestyle practices to address diverse ailments, including epilepsy and seizures in kids.

UNDERSTANDING THE AYURVEDIC SYSTEM OF MEDICINE:
According to Ayurveda, epilepsy and seizures in youngsters are considered illnesses of the "Vata" dosha, which symbolizes the energy of movement and communication in the body. Imbalances in Vata dosha may lead to irregular nerve impulses and abnormalities in the brain, resulting in seizures. Ayurveda tries to restore balance to the Vata dosha and soothe the nervous system to minimize the frequency and severity of seizures.

AYURVEDIC HERBS AND TREATMENTS FOR EPILEPSY MANAGEMENT:
Ashwagandha (Withania somnifera): Ashwagandha is an adaptogenic herb that helps decrease stress and anxiety, which may be triggering factors for seizures. It contains neuroprotective qualities and helps the general health of the nervous system.

Brahmi (Bacopa monnieri): Brahmi is recognized for its cognitive-enhancing effects. It helps boost memory, focus, and general brain function. It also functions as an anticonvulsant and may aid in lowering the frequency of seizures.

Shankhpushpi (Convolvulus pluricaulis): Shankhpushpi is excellent for the neurological system. It helps alleviate restlessness, anxiety, and impatience and promotes tranquillity and mental clarity.

Jatamansi (Nardostachys jatamansi): Jatamansi is regarded as an effective herb for soothing the nervous system. It aids in lowering tension, anxiety, and sleeplessness, and may be effective in treating epilepsy and seizures.

In addition to these medicines, Ayurveda stresses the need for lifestyle alterations and dietary changes for epilepsy treatment in youngsters. This may involve practicing frequent meditation and yoga, having a consistent daily schedule, avoiding triggers like excessive screen time and late nights, and following a balanced diet that includes fresh fruits, vegetables, whole grains, and healthy fats.

COMBINING AYURVEDA WITH CONVENTIONAL EPILEPSY TREATMENTS:
It's vital to emphasize that Ayurveda should not be regarded as a sole therapy for epilepsy in youngsters. It may be used as a

complementary technique with standard medical treatments provided by healthcare specialists. Ayurvedic medicines and therapies may aid in controlling symptoms, lowering the frequency of seizures, and increasing general well-being. However, it is vital to consult with a skilled Ayurvedic practitioner and work in partnership with a pediatric neurologist to build an integrated treatment plan that meets the individual requirements of the kid.

When integrating Ayurveda with standard epilepsy therapies, communication and collaboration between healthcare practitioners are crucial. The pediatric neurologist should be informed about the Ayurvedic remedies being employed, and any changes in the child's health or treatment plan should be reported to both practitioners.

It's crucial to note that every kid is unique, and the success of Ayurvedic therapy may vary. Close monitoring of the child's symptoms, frequent check-ups with healthcare experts, and open communication among all concerned parties are critical for the optimum treatment of epilepsy in youngsters.

In summary, Ayurveda provides a comprehensive approach to controlling epilepsy and seizures in kids by resolving imbalances in the body and soothing the nervous system. It comprises the use of certain herbs, lifestyle alterations, and dietary changes. However, it should be used in combination with traditional medical therapies and under the advice of experienced practitioners to achieve the greatest results for the child's health.

INTEGRATING COMPLEMENTARY AND ALTERNATIVE TREATMENTS - Developing an integrated approach to epilepsy management

- Communicating with healthcare doctors about complementary therapies
- Creating a specific treatment plan for your kid

Epilepsy is a neurological condition marked by recurring seizures. While traditional medical therapies such as antiepileptic medications (AEDs) remain the primary strategy for controlling epilepsy in children, many parents and caregivers seek alternative choices to supplement their child's therapy. Complementary and alternative treatments (CATs) are non-mainstream therapies that may be utilized with traditional medicine to give a comprehensive approach to epilepsy care.

Integrating CATs into a complete treatment strategy might possibly benefit the overall well-being and seizure management in children. Here, we will discuss the many parts of constructing an integrated strategy for epilepsy management for kids, speaking with healthcare professionals about complementary therapies, and creating a specific treatment plan for your child.

DEVELOPING AN INTEGRATED APPROACH TO EPILEPSY MANAGEMENT:
Consult with a healthcare team: It is vital to consult a team of healthcare providers specialized in treating juvenile epilepsy, including neurologists, epileptologists, pediatricians, and other specialists. They may give advice on implementing CATs into your child's treatment plan while assuring safety and optimizing the overall care.

Understand the traditional treatment: It is crucial to have a complete grasp of the conventional therapy your kid is presently taking, such as particular antiepileptic drugs, their dose, and any adverse effects. This information will help you discover places where CATs may enhance the present treatment approach.

Research CAT options: Educate yourself on different CATs available for epilepsy treatment, such as dietary interventions (ketogenic diet, modified Atkins diet), herbal medicines, acupuncture, mindfulness-based therapies, and biofeedback. Understand the data supporting their effectiveness, possible hazards, and any contraindications.

Evaluate the compatibility: Assess the compatibility of CATs with your child's general health, medical history, and present therapies. Some CATs may have interactions with particular drugs, while others may not be acceptable for children with specific disorders. It is vital to address these factors with your healthcare team to guarantee the safety and efficacy of incorporating CATs.

Consider the kid's preferences: Involve your youngster, to the degree feasible, in decision-making on CATs. Their willingness to contribute may boost the effectiveness of the treatment plan and empower them to take control of their health.

COMMUNICATING WITH HEALTHCARE PROVIDERS ABOUT COMPLEMENTARY TREATMENTS:

Open and honest communication: Establish a relationship of trust and open communication with your child's healthcare staff. Inform them about your interest in investigating CATs and your study on alternative choices. This interaction will allow an educated debate, enabling healthcare practitioners to share their knowledge and concerns and ensure that everyone is on the same page.

Share information: Provide your healthcare team with accurate and detailed information on the particular CATs you are considering.

Share any relevant research or studies supporting their usage in epilepsy treatment. This information will aid healthcare practitioners in analyzing the possible advantages and hazards and making educated choices in the best interest of their kid.

Ask for expert guidance: Request your healthcare team's feedback on the CATs you are contemplating. They may give insights based on their medical knowledge and experience, helping you analyze the appropriateness, safety, and possible combinations with current medications.

Regular follow-ups: Establish a timetable for regular check-ins with your healthcare team to monitor your child's development, address any changes or concerns, and assess the effect of the integrated treatment plan. These follow-ups will assist ensure that the CATs are successfully incorporated into the overall management and altered as appropriate.

CREATING A PERSONALIZED EPILEPSY AND SEIZURES TREATMENT PLAN:

Individualize the treatment strategy: Work with your healthcare team to build a customized treatment plan that includes CATs suited to your child's individual requirements, medical history, and seizure patterns. This strategy should examine aspects such as the kind of epilepsy, frequency and severity of seizures, any known triggers, and your child's general health and preferences.

Set reasonable objectives: Collaborate with your healthcare team to develop realistic goals for your child's treatment, taking into consideration the possible advantages and limits of both conventional and complementary therapies. These aims may include lowering seizure frequency and intensity, enhancing general well-being and quality of life, minimizing adverse effects of drugs, and fostering cognitive growth and social integration.

collaboration among healthcare providers: If your kid gets CATs from different healthcare professionals, promote excellent communication and collaboration among them. This cooperation will eliminate any conflicts or duplications and maximize the integration of CATs into the overall treatment plan.

Monitor and document outcomes: Keep a record of your child's seizure frequency, severity, and any changes in their general well-being. Regularly share this information with your healthcare team to analyze the success of the integrated treatment plan. This record will allow modifications to be made as required and give vital insights for future decision-making.

Remember that incorporating CATs into the therapy of epilepsy and seizures for youngsters should always be done under the advice and supervision of healthcare experts. While CATs might give extra assistance, they should never replace or compromise traditional medical therapies. The integrated approach should stress safety, evidence-based procedures, and the best interest of the child, delivering a complete and holistic care strategy for epilepsy.

QUESTIONS PARENTS WITH KIDS WHO HAVE EPILEPSY & SEIZURES CAN ASK THEIR HEALTHCARE PROVIDER

- What type of epilepsy or seizures does my child/ I have?
- What are the common triggers for seizures in children/ adults with epilepsy?

- What are the potential risks and complications associated with epilepsy or seizures?
- What medications are typically prescribed for epilepsy management, and what are their potential side effects?
- Are there any specific precautions or lifestyle changes my child/ I need to follow to manage epilepsy?
- Are there any dietary restrictions or recommendations that can help in managing seizures?
- Are there any specific warning signs or symptoms that indicate a seizure is about to occur?
- How often should my child/ I have follow-up appointments to monitor epilepsy and adjust treatment if necessary?
- Are there any specific tests or diagnostic procedures that need to be performed regularly to assess epilepsy management?

- What are the potential long-term effects of epilepsy on my child's/ my development and overall health?
- Are there any known genetic factors associated with epilepsy that I should be aware of?
- Are there any specific safety measures or precautions I should take at home, school, or during recreational activities to prevent injuries during seizures?
- Are there any alternative treatment options or complementary therapies that can be used alongside traditional medications for epilepsy management?
- What is the scientific evidence supporting the effectiveness of alternative treatments for epilepsy and seizures?
- Are there any risks or potential interactions between alternative treatments and traditional epilepsy medications?

- How do alternative treatments for epilepsy work? Are there any specific mechanisms of action or theories behind their effectiveness?
- Are there any reputable clinical trials or research studies exploring the use of alternative treatments for epilepsy in children/ adults?
- What are the potential benefits and drawbacks of using alternative treatments for epilepsy in children/ adults?
- Can alternative treatments completely replace traditional epilepsy medications, or are they typically used as complementary approaches?
- Are there any specific alternative treatments that have shown promising results in managing epilepsy in children/ adults?
- How do you assess the safety and reliability of alternative treatment providers or practitioners?

- Are there any specific dietary supplements or herbal remedies that have been found to be effective in reducing seizure frequency?
- Are there any lifestyle changes, such as stress management techniques or sleep hygiene practices, that can help in seizure management?
- What are the potential costs associated with alternative treatments for epilepsy, and are they covered by insurance?
- Are there any support groups or resources available for parents of children with epilepsy or individuals with epilepsy looking to explore alternative treatments?
- How can I monitor and track the effectiveness of alternative treatments for epilepsy in my child/ myself?
- Are there any potential interactions between alternative treatments and other medications or medical conditions my child/ I have?

- Can you provide references or recommend reputable sources of information on alternative treatments for epilepsy?
- Are there any known risks or side effects associated with specific alternative treatments for epilepsy?
- How does stress management and mental health impact seizure frequency and overall epilepsy management?
- Are there any specific relaxation techniques or therapies that have shown to be beneficial for epilepsy management?
- What role does sleep play in epilepsy management, and are there any specific sleep-related recommendations?
- How does nutrition and hydration impact seizures and overall epilepsy management?
- Are there any specific exercises or physical activities that should be

avoided or encouraged for individuals with epilepsy?

- Can changes in hormonal levels affect seizures, and are there any specific considerations for puberty or menopause?
- Are there any environmental factors or triggers that could worsen seizures in children/ adults with epilepsy?
- Are there any technological devices or apps that can help monitor seizures and provide assistance during an episode?
- Can epilepsy affect cognitive abilities or learning capabilities, and are there any interventions or accommodations available?
- Are there any specific precautions or recommendations for individuals with epilepsy regarding driving or operating machinery?
- How does epilepsy affect social interactions and relationships, and are

there any strategies for managing these challenges?

- Can epilepsy be outgrown or go into remission? What factors contribute to a better prognosis?
- Are there any specific measures or plans in place for emergencies or seizure clusters?
- Can stress reduction techniques, such as biofeedback or meditation, help in managing epilepsy symptoms?
- Are there any specific vitamins or minerals that are beneficial for individuals with epilepsy?
- Are there any potential alternative therapies, such as acupuncture or chiropractic care, that could complement traditional epilepsy treatments?
- Can the use of medical marijuana or CBD products be considered as alternative treatments for epilepsy?

- Are there any specific relaxation techniques or therapies suitable for young children with epilepsy?
- What are the potential benefits and drawbacks of using ketogenic diets or modified Atkins diets in epilepsy management?
- How can I differentiate between reliable and unreliable sources of information on complementary and alternative treatments for epilepsy?
- Are there any ongoing research studies or clinical trials investigating alternative treatments for epilepsy that my child/ I can participate in?

CHAPTER 4

<u>The Menu for Success: Exploring Dietary Options for Childhood Epilepsy</u>

IMPORTANCE OF DIET IN MANAGING EPILEPSY AND SEIZURES

Managing epilepsy and seizures in children involves a comprehensive strategy that includes medical therapy, lifestyle adjustments, and nutritional considerations. While medicine is frequently the main treatment strategy, research has shown that nutrition has a key role in treating epilepsy and lowering the frequency and severity of seizures, especially in youngsters. In reality, for some children with epilepsy, dietary changes may be an effective alternative or supplemental therapy.

Several particular diets have been designed and found to be useful in treating epilepsy in youngsters. These include the ketogenic diet, modified Atkins diet, and low glycemic index therapy. These diets are heavy in fat and low in carbs and protein, which puts the body's metabolism into a state of ketosis. Ketosis is a metabolic state in which the body depends on fat for fuel instead of glucose, resulting in the generation of ketones. The presence of ketones in the blood has been connected with a decrease in seizure activity.

The ketogenic diet, in particular, has demonstrated exceptional efficacy in lowering seizures in children with epilepsy. It requires a rigorous regulation of the ratio of fat to carbohydrates and protein in the diet. Typically, the ketogenic diet consists of a ratio of 3:1 or 4:1 (fat to combined protein and carbs). This indicates that roughly 90% of the daily calorie intake comes from fat sources, with the remaining 10% distributed between protein and carbs. The modified Atkins diet is less stringent but still supports a greater consumption of fats and a lower intake of carbs.

The reasons underlying the success of these diets in treating epilepsy are not yet completely understood. However, various explanations have been offered. One idea is that ketones created during the breakdown of fat may have an anticonvulsant impact on the brain. Another idea indicates that the diet changes neurotransmitter activity, regulating brain excitability and minimizing the probability of seizures. Additionally, the ketogenic diet may have anti-inflammatory and antioxidant benefits, which might potentially contribute to its good influence on seizure management.

It's vital to remember that establishing a specific diet for epilepsy involves constant supervision by a healthcare expert, often a licensed dietitian or a neurologist specializing in epilepsy. They will analyze the child's nutritional requirements, give assistance with meal planning, and monitor the child's development. Regular follow-up visits are necessary to verify the diet is being correctly adopted and changed as required.

While the ketogenic diet and other dietary therapies have demonstrated considerable advantages in treating epilepsy and lowering seizures in children, it's crucial to note that not all children will react similarly. Each kid is unique, and what works for one may not work for another. Some children may receive a total cessation of seizures, while others may find a reduction in seizure frequency or intensity.

In certain circumstances, the diet may not have a substantial influence on seizure management at all. Therefore, it is crucial to work closely with healthcare specialists to determine the best appropriate solution for each unique kid.

In conclusion, nutrition has a key role in treating epilepsy and seizures in children. While drugs are frequently the main treatment option, dietary treatments such as the ketogenic diet have shown promise in lowering seizure activity.

These specific diets may function by modifying the body's metabolism, regulating brain excitability, and offering anti-inflammatory and antioxidant benefits. However, it is vital to obtain help from healthcare specialists when contemplating establishing a customized diet for epilepsy to guarantee correct monitoring, nutritional balance, and efficacy for the kid.

EXPLORING DIETARY APPROACHES
- Ketogenic diet: Principles, advantages, and problems
- Sample meal ideas and recipes for a ketogenic diet

- **Modified Atkins diet: Principles, advantages, and problems**
- **Sample meal ideas and recipes for a modified Atkins diet**
- **Low glycemic index diet: Principles, advantages, and problems**
- **Sample meal ideas and dishes for a low glycemic index diet**

KETOGENIC DIET FOR SEIZURES AND EPILEPSY: Principles, Benefits, and Challenges

The ketogenic diet is a high-fat, low-carbohydrate, and moderate-protein diet that has been used for decades as a treatment method for seizures and epilepsy, especially in children who have not reacted well to standard drugs. The diet works by establishing a state of ketosis, when the body largely depends on ketones, a byproduct of fat breakdown, for energy instead of glucose.

Principles:

1. High-fat consumption: The ketogenic diet involves a large increase in dietary fat intake, generally representing roughly 70-90% of total daily calories.

2. Low carbohydrate intake: Carbohydrates are tightly restricted, often confined to 20-50 grams per day or roughly 5-10% of total daily calories.

3. Moderate protein intake: Protein consumption is reduced to roughly 1 gram per kilogram of body weight or about 10-20% of total daily calories.

4. Strict monitoring: The diet must be closely controlled, with exact ratios of fat, carbs, and protein maintained in each meal to establish and sustain ketosis.

Benefits:

1. Seizure control: The major advantage of the ketogenic diet is its success in lowering seizure frequency and intensity, especially in children who have not reacted well to antiepileptic medicines.

2. Reduced drug dependence: Some children may be able to lessen or eliminate their dependency on antiepileptic medicines while on the ketogenic diet, possibly lowering medication side effects.

3. Cognitive improvements: There is evidence to show that the ketogenic diet may enhance cognitive performance and behavior in children with epilepsy.

Challenges:

1. strong adherence: Following a ketogenic diet needs strong commitment and discipline, which may be tough, particularly for children and their families.

2. Nutritional deficits: The restricted food options in the diet may lead to possible nutritional deficiencies. Careful supplementation and monitoring of vitamin and mineral consumption are needed.

3. Social effect: The ketogenic diet may influence a child's social life since it frequently prohibits the eating of popular items like bread, pasta, and sweets. This

might make it tough for youngsters to engage in social gatherings involving eating.

SAMPLE MEAL IDEAS AND RECIPES FOR A KETOGENIC DIET FOR KIDS:

1. Breakfast: Scrambled eggs cooked in butter with avocado slices and bacon.

2. Lunch: Chicken salad prepared with mayonnaise, chopped chicken, celery, and walnuts served on a bed of lettuce.

3. Snack: Cheese slices with cucumber or celery sticks.

4. Dinner: Grilled salmon with roasted broccoli and cauliflower drizzled with olive oil.

5. Dessert: Sugar-free raspberry chia pudding cooked with coconut milk and sweetened with a sugar replacement like stevia.

MODIFIED ATKINS DIET FOR EPILEPSY AND SEIZURES: Principles, Benefits, and Challenges

The Modified Atkins Diet (MAD) is another dietary treatment used for epilepsy and seizures, which is less restrictive than the standard ketogenic diet. It follows a similar low-carbohydrate approach but allows for somewhat more protein and carbohydrate consumption.

Principles:

1. Low carbohydrate intake: The Modified Atkins Diet limits carbs to a maximum of 10-20 grams per day during the beginning phases, progressively rising to roughly 40-60 grams per day.

2. High fat intake: The bulk of calories come from fat, totalling roughly 60-70% of total daily calories.

3. Adequate protein intake: Protein consumption is liberalized and not rigorously limited as in the ketogenic diet but maintained at a moderate level.

Benefits:

1. Seizure control: The Modified Atkins Diet has proven effectiveness in lowering seizure frequency and severity in children with epilepsy.

2. Simplicity and flexibility:

Compared to the ketogenic diet, the Modified Atkins Diet is easier to execute and provides greater nutritional flexibility, making it more practical for certain families.

Challenges:

1. Limited food choices: While the Modified Atkins Diet gives more freedom than the ketogenic diet, there are still limits on high-carbohydrate items, which may be problematic for youngsters.

2. Adherence and monitoring: Consistent adherence to the diet and frequent monitoring of carbohydrate consumption may be hard and need continuing assistance and direction.

3. Potential adverse effects: Some children may develop gastrointestinal difficulties,

such as constipation or diarrhea, owing to the high-fat content of the diet.

SAMPLE MEAL IDEAS AND RECIPES FOR A MODIFIED ATKINS DIET:

1. Breakfast: Almond flour pancakes topped with sugar-free syrup and a side of scrambled eggs.
2. Lunch: Lettuce wraps loaded with deli meat, cheese, and avocado slices.
3. Snack: Celery sticks with almond butter or cream cheese.
4. Dinner: Grilled chicken breast with steamed veggies sautéed in butter.
5. Dessert: Sugar-free peanut butter cookies prepared with almond flour and sweetened with a sugar replacement like erythritol.

LOW GLYCEMIC INDEX DIET FOR EPILEPSY AND SEIZURES: Principles, Benefits, and Challenges

The low glycemic index (GI) diet focuses on ingesting carbohydrates with a lower glycemic index, meaning they have a slower and more gradual influence on blood sugar levels. This technique tries to give a continuous flow of glucose into circulation, reducing blood sugar spikes and maintaining more consistent energy levels.

Principles:

1. Low glycemic index foods: The low GI diet emphasizes foods that have a low glycemic index, such as whole grains, legumes, non-starchy vegetables, and low-sugar fruits.

2. Balanced macronutrient ratios: The diet strives for a balanced consumption of carbs, proteins, and fats without any excessive limits.

3. Fiber-rich meals: Incorporating high-fiber foods helps slow down digestion and absorption, further helping to stabilize blood sugar levels.

Benefits:

1. Stable blood sugar levels: By concentrating on low GI foods, the diet

helps maintain more stable blood sugar levels throughout the day, which may contribute to general well-being.

2. Improved energy and satiety: Foods with a lower glycemic index tend to give longer-lasting energy and enhance feelings of fullness, lowering the probability of energy crashes or overeating.

3. Balanced nutrition: Unlike the ketogenic and Modified Atkins diets, the low GI diet does not drastically limit any macronutrients, allowing for a more diversified and nutritionally balanced approach.

Challenges:

1. Individual response: The glycemic index may vary across people, and specific variables like meal combinations and cooking techniques might alter it. Finding the correct combination of low-GI meals for optimum outcomes may need some experimenting.

2. Food availability and choices: While many low GI foods are easily accessible, it may still need careful planning and selection to include them into a child's diet.

3. Monitoring and education: Understanding the glycemic index and how to make optimal meal choices involves education and constant monitoring.

SAMPLE MEAL IDEAS AND RECIPES FOR A LOW GLYCEMIC INDEX DIET:

1. Breakfast: Overnight oats prepared with rolled oats, unsweetened almond milk, chia seeds, and berries.

2. Lunch: Quinoa salad with mixed veggies, grilled chicken, and a vinaigrette dressing.

3. Snack: Apple slices with almond butter.

4. Dinner: Baked salmon with roasted sweet potatoes and steamed broccoli.

5. Dessert: Greek yogurt with mixed berries and a sprinkling of chopped nuts.

Note: It's vital to check with a healthcare practitioner or a certified dietitian before initiating any dietary intervention for seizures or epilepsy in children. They may give tailored instruction, assure nutritional adequacy, and monitor the child's development.

MEAL PLANNING AND Nutritional Considerations
- Key nutrition for children with epilepsy
- Portion sizes and calorie needs
- Balancing macronutrients (carbohydrates, protein, and fat)
- Micronutrient-rich foods to include in the diet
- Managing food limitations and allergies
- Tips for efficient meal planning and preparation
While medicine is the main therapy for epilepsy, appropriate diet and meal planning may play a key role in controlling the illness and minimizing the frequency

and severity of seizures. Here, we will discuss important nutrients, portion sizes, macronutrient balance, micronutrient-rich foods, handling limits and allergies, and strategies for effective meal planning and preparation for children with epilepsy and seizures.

KEY NUTRIENTS FOR CHILDREN WITH EPILEPSY:
Certain nutrients have been discovered to be useful for children with epilepsy and seizures. These include:

Omega-3 Fatty Acids: Found in fatty fish, flaxseeds, and walnuts, omega-3 fatty acids have anti-inflammatory qualities and may boost brain function.

Vitamin D: Adequate vitamin D levels have been connected with decreased seizure frequency. Good sources of vitamin D include fortified dairy products, fatty fish, and sunshine exposure.

Vitamin B6: Vitamin B6 is involved in the synthesis of neurotransmitters. Foods high in vitamin B6 include chicken, fish, whole grains, bananas, and potatoes.

Magnesium: Magnesium has been proven to have anticonvulsant properties. Good sources of magnesium include green leafy vegetables, nuts, seeds, and whole grains.

PORTION SIZES AND CALORIE REQUIREMENTS:
Portion sizes and calorie needs for children with epilepsy and seizures are comparable to those of children without the illness. It is crucial to ensure that youngsters acquire appropriate energy to sustain growth and development. Calorie demands might vary based on the child's age, weight, height, activity level, and general health. Consulting with a trained dietitian may assist estimate optimal calorie needs for an individual kid.

BALANCING MACRONUTRIENTS FOR CHILDREN WITH EPILEPSY AND SEIZURES:
Maintaining a balanced intake of macronutrients is vital for general health and seizure treatment. While the precise ratio may vary based on the child's unique requirements, a diet rich in healthy fats and low in carbs has been demonstrated to be helpful for certain children with epilepsy.

This method, known as the ketogenic diet, encourages the creation of ketones, which may help decrease seizure activity. However, it is crucial to engage closely with a healthcare practitioner and a certified dietitian while following a ketogenic diet, since it involves constant monitoring and supervision.

Micronutrient-Rich Foods to Include in the Diet of Children with Epilepsy and Seizures: In addition to vital nutrients, it is necessary to incorporate a range of micronutrient-rich foods in the diet of children with epilepsy and seizures. These include:

Fruits and Vegetables: Rich in vitamins, minerals, and antioxidants, fruits and vegetables should constitute a large portion of the child's diet. Aim for a colorful assortment to provide a broad spectrum of nutrients.

Whole Grains: Whole grains contain critical minerals and fiber. Opt for whole-grain bread, pasta, rice, and cereals instead of processed grains.

Lean Protein: Choose lean sources of protein such as chicken, fish, lentils, and tofu. Protein is necessary for development, repair, and general health.

Managing Food Restrictions and Allergies for Kids with Epilepsy and Seizures:
Some children with epilepsy may have extra dietary restrictions or allergies that need to

be taken into account. It is crucial to engage with a healthcare team, including a qualified dietitian, to design a meal plan that satisfies the child's nutritional requirements while meeting any unique dietary restrictions or allergies. This may include identifying adequate substitutes and ensuring that the child's food stays balanced and healthy.

TIPS FOR SUCCESSFUL MEAL PLANNING AND PREPARATION:
Involve the kid: Encourage the youngster to participate in meal planning and preparation. This may assist enhance their interest in and acceptance of different meals and tastes.

Create a routine: Establish regular meal and snack times to help regulate blood sugar levels and reduce hunger-related triggers for seizures.

Keep a food diary: Keep note of the child's meals, snacks, and seizure activity. This may help discover possible triggers or trends and aid in fine-tuning the diet plan.

Be careful of drugs: Some medications used to control epilepsy may interfere with particular foods or necessitate alterations in the timing of meals. Consult with the child's healthcare team for advice.

Stay hydrated: Proper hydration is vital for general health. Encourage the youngster to drink an appropriate quantity of water throughout the day.

Seek assistance: Joining support groups or interacting with other parents of children with epilepsy may give useful insights, advice, and emotional support.

In conclusion, appropriate meal planning and nutrition are crucial components in controlling epilepsy and seizures in children. By ensuring a balanced intake of key nutrients, considering portion sizes and calorie requirements, balancing macronutrients, incorporating micronutrient-rich foods, managing restrictions and allergies, and following the tips for successful meal planning and preparation, parents and caregivers can support their child's overall health and well-being while minimizing the impact of seizures. Always consult with healthcare experts, especially registered dietitians, for individualized counsel based on the child's unique requirements.

IMPLEMENTING A DIET FOR CHILDREN WITH EPILEPSY
- Getting started with a new diet
- Tracking and monitoring progress
- Working with healthcare professionals and dietitians
- Addressing frequent issues and setbacks
- Supporting the child's psychological well-being

When it comes to controlling epilepsy and seizures in children, nutrition has a key role in lowering the frequency and severity of seizures. Certain dietary treatments, such as the ketogenic diet and modified Atkins diet, have been demonstrated to be useful in controlling epilepsy.

However, creating and maintaining a customized diet for children with epilepsy involves careful planning, monitoring, and coordination with healthcare specialists. In this post, we will cover the numerous elements of creating a diet for children with epilepsy and seizures.

GETTING STARTED WITH A NEW DIET:
Implementing a new diet for a kid with epilepsy and seizures should begin with a full review by a healthcare practitioner or a qualified dietitian with experience in epilepsy. They may examine the child's medical history, seizure patterns, current

food habits, and any other pertinent aspects. Based on this evaluation, they may propose a suitable nutritional regimen, such as the ketogenic diet or modified Atkins diet.

The shift to a specific diet should be gradual and well-planned. It is necessary to educate the child's caregivers, including parents and other family members, on the principles and needs of the diet. They need to understand the suggested dietary choices, quantity amounts, meal planning, and any side effects. It may be beneficial to study resources such as cookbooks, online forums, and support groups specialized in epilepsy and diet.

TRACKING AND MONITORING THE PROGRESS OF DIET:
Regular monitoring of the child's development on the diet is vital for assessing its efficacy and making any modifications. This may be done via numerous means, including keeping a

seizure journal, documenting the child's weight and development, and undergoing frequent medical check-ups.

Keeping a seizure journal helps document the frequency, length, and severity of seizures before and after beginning the diet. This information may give useful insights into the efficacy of the diet and aid healthcare practitioners in making suitable alterations.

Monitoring the child's weight and development is vital, since certain diet adjustments may impact nutrient intake and growth trends. Regular check-ups with the child's healthcare team may ensure that any possible nutritional deficiencies are recognized and handled immediately.

WORKING WITH HEALTHCARE PROFESSIONALS AND DIETITIANS OF CHILDREN WITH EPILEPSY AND SEIZURES:

Collaboration with healthcare specialists and qualified dietitians specialized in epilepsy is required during the administration of the diet. They may give continuing supervision, assess the child's development, and make modifications to the diet as required.

Healthcare providers may undertake frequent examinations to monitor the child's reaction to the diet, alter medicines if appropriate, and address any concerns or adverse effects. Registered dietitians may create tailored meal plans, propose optimal food choices, provide direction on reaching nutritional needs, and handle any issues relating to the diet.

It is vital to keep open contact with the healthcare staff and seek their help whenever required. Regular follow-ups with healthcare experts and dietitians may ensure that the child's food is adequately regulated and adjusted for the greatest seizure management.

ADDRESSING COMMON CHALLENGES AND SETBACKS REGARDING DIET:
Implementing a specific diet for children with epilepsy and seizures might bring various problems and setbacks. Some typical obstacles include dietary limits, difficulty in obtaining adequate food substitutes, social isolation, and lack of compliance.

To address these problems, it is crucial to include the whole family in meal planning and preparation, making it a joint endeavor. Exploring inventive recipes, getting help from online forums or support groups, and connecting with other families experiencing similar issues may give a great support system.

Encouraging social contacts and informing people about the child's nutritional requirements might help lessen feelings of isolation. Communication with teachers, school workers, and caregivers outside the immediate family is crucial to ensure the child's diet is respected and accommodated.

Supporting the Child's Psychological Well-being while they suffer Epilepsy and Seizures:
Living with epilepsy and sticking to a particular diet might influence a child's psychological well-being. It is crucial to give emotional support, create a good self-image, and educate the youngster on their illness and dietary needs.

Encouraging open dialogues about epilepsy and diet may help the youngster better understand their condition and feel more powerful. Recognizing and praising their successes and milestones, both connected to the diet and in other aspects of their life helps increase their self-esteem.

Engaging in age-appropriate activities, hobbies, and social connections may contribute to a well-rounded and satisfying existence, helping the kid deal with the problems of epilepsy.

Conclusion:
Implementing a diet for children with epilepsy and seizures involves careful planning, continual monitoring, and coordination with healthcare experts and nutritionists. By adopting a planned strategy, addressing obstacles proactively, and giving emotional support, the child's journey with epilepsy may be effectively controlled, leading to increased seizure control and overall well-being.